6 WAYS TO LOSE BELLY FAT WITHOUT EXERCISE!

JJ Smith

6 WAYS TO LOSE BELLY FAT WITHOUT EXERCISE!

by JJ Smith

Published by Adiva Publishing
12138 Central Ave, Ste. 391
Mitchellville, MD 20721
For more information, see www.JJSmithOnline.com.

Library of Congress Cataloging-in-Publication Data

Smith, JJ

6 Ways to Lose Belly Fat Without Exercise! /JJ Smith, First Edition

1. Health/Diet 2. Weight Loss 3. Women's Health and Wellness

ISBN: 978-0-9823018-8-3

Testimonials for
"6 Ways to Lose Belly Fat Without Exercise!"

"So far, I have lost 4 lbs and 2 inches off my belly in the first week! I am so excited. I want to thank you for all your info and caring enough to share it with us. Thank you so much!!!"
—Carolyn S.

"I dropped 3 inches in my waist the first 10 days!!!"
—Vanessa B.

"I have been following *6 Ways to Lose Belly Fat Without Exercise* since Sept 24th, and in 3 WEEKS, I have lost 5 INCHES from my waist/belly area!!!! Slimmer abs are within me!! I am beginning to lose the belly fat!!! I almost couldn't go to sleep for dreaming of my future . . . And how my life and body are transforming into a better me. I just had to share, just couldn't help it. Thank you!! It's truly working for me! And I honestly have not been working out at all, and I'm still getting these amazing results!!!"
—Debra P.

"I have lost so much belly fat . . . I lost close to 5 inches in my stomach area in just one month. I'm so, so happy about that; my sister just doesn't believe that I haven't worked out, not once."
—Clarisse J.

"I'm 44 years old and, like most men, I have always dreamed of having a six-pack. I have worked out off and on my entire life but never could achieve that elusive six-pack until I discovered JJ's program to lose belly fat without exercise. I lost 14 pounds in 3 weeks and am constantly looking at or taking pictures of my abs. My abs look better now than they did when I was 21 years old!"
—Tyler J.

"This has truly been life-changing for me. I am an avid gym rat but could not seem to get rid of my belly; 3 months on your program and I can see the abs forming in my pictures, and I couldn't be happier. So . . . all I can say is thank you, thank you, thank you!"

—Moe B.

"I am 6 pounds down—3 inches lost in the belly area and 2 inches in the waist area. I am really happy with my results and appreciate the helpful recipes. My metabolism is back up and I feel really good!"

—Christie C.

"I went from a 41 waistline to a 38, losing 3 inches in the first 3 weeks."

—Geraldine S.

"I purchased *6 Ways to Lose Belly Fat Without Exercise* seven days ago, and I've lost two inches off my waist in ONE WEEK. As far as the BELLY FAT . . . It is almost completely GONE!!!"

—Lashell

Table of Contents

Important Note to Readers

The information contained in this book is for your education. It is not intended to diagnose, treat, or cure any medical condition or dispense medical advice. If you decide to follow my plan, you should seek the advice and counsel of a licensed health professional and then use your own judgment.

It is important to obtain proper medical advice before you make any decisions about nutrition, diet, supplements, or other health-related issues that are discussed in this book. Neither the author nor the publisher is qualified to provide medical, financial, or psychological advice or services. The reader should consult an appropriate healthcare professional before heeding any of the advice given in this book.

Preface

I am a nutritionist, a certified weight-loss expert, author of the #1 bestseller *Lose Weight Without Dieting or Working Out*, and creator of the Detox-Eat-Move (DEM) System. I help people lose weight without dieting and working out so they can get their sexy back!

Every day, I get asked the same question: "How can I get rid of belly fat?" I totally understand why! I used to be so frustrated with my belly. I looked like I was about three months' pregnant and wore big baggy shirts to cover it. I have been where you are today. But then I spent years figuring out what was causing my belly fat and learned how to get rid of it for good. My goal for writing this book is to teach you how to get rid of your belly fat once and for all!

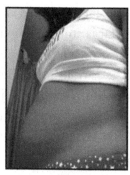 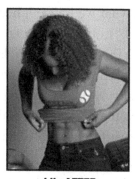

JJ's BEFORE   **JJ's AFTER**

When I went on the *Steve Harvey Morning Show*, I showed them before-and-after photos of my belly that I had taken with my cell phone. They were amazed by the difference and suggested I share the pictures on my website. Well, as struggling with weight is deeply personal, I couldn't bring myself to post them then. However, my clients will tell you that I do know what works and works very well for getting rid of belly fat. But for the sake of convincing any doubters, I will finally share the photos so that readers can see the results of these six strategies that helped me get rid of my belly fat without exercise.

I must say I'm so excited to write this book because you have asked for it. Every single day someone asks me how to get rid of belly fat. I have answered that by creating the most comprehensive program ever created on how to get rid of belly fat once and for all. Yes, it's possible to lose belly fat WITHOUT exercise, without sit-ups or crunches, without long boring cardio workouts, without ab belts or gadgets—and no fad diets!

I want to tell you a little secret that weight loss experts know. It is really important to understand this concept. Here's what we know: There is body fat and there is what is called "stubborn body fat." Belly fat is stubborn body fat because this type of fat sticks to the stomach and generally doesn't respond very well to exercise or traditional dieting. Generally speaking, eating healthy and being physically active will help you lose body fat. But that "stubborn body fat" is a different kind of fat, and that's what belly fat is.

Now I have some bad news about belly fat. Most people do not know that belly fat is actually the most dangerous fat on the body. Why? Because of where it's located around the delicate organs, it has the potential to destroy good health, or worse yet, kill you. Because belly fat resides within striking distance of your heart, liver, and other delicate organs, it is to blame for many health conditions. According to a 2006 study published in the journal *Obesity*, belly fat (also known as visceral fat) is a significant predictor of early death. In other words, visceral fat/belly fat means you have an increased risk for a shortened life. Even if you were to remove visceral fat via liposuction, allowing you to look better on the outside, that would do little to improve your overall health because the dangers of visceral fat would still exist for you.

The good news is that I have created a comprehensive program with six ways you can get rid of belly fat/visceral fat, and none of them involves exercise.

One reason I don't focus on exercises to flatten the stomach is because we already know this advice and have heard it over and over again. How many fitness trainers do we need to tell us that we should do sit-ups and ab crunches to lose belly fat? We've heard it, yet so many of us are still struggling to get those slim, sexy abs that we desire.

Now do ab crunches and sit-ups work? Fitness experts tell me that they do. But I don't do any of these sorts of exercises and neither do most of my clients, yet we've all achieved a flatter stomach and slimmer waistline. I do not teach things that I don't do myself. I'd rather leave that to the fitness trainers. If you choose to do ab crunches, go right ahead. They may even help. But they're not required in order to get results with this program.

I have personally used these six strategies I'm going to share in this book and have successfully gotten rid of my belly fat! And I'm so happy about that. In the beginning of this book, I shared a few of the testimonials from others who have had success losing belly fat with these six strategies. And you, too, can get a slimmer waistline and get rid of belly fat without exercise. I will hold your hand and show you step-by-step how to do this.

To be responsible, I will give you my public service announcement about exercise: We should all get as much exercise as possible because it's good for overall health. I am definitely not against exercise. It would be irresponsible of me to discourage exercise. I always encourage people to get more active and to get moving—it's great for cardio health.

I want you to understand that everyone has flat abs underneath once you get rid of the fat. So, we focus on burning that fat away so you can naturally reveal your sexy, slimmer abs. They are already under there, we just have to burn that belly fat away!

It is possible to lose belly fat without sit-ups, crunches, long cardio workouts, or ab belts and other gadgets. And without going on a fad diet. You really have a choice today. You can invest in you, not just because belly fat is dangerously unhealthy, but so you can have those slimmer, sexier, healthier abs you desire.

Please try the program and then write me and let me know how much belly fat you've lost. I look forward to hearing your success story!

JJ Smith

Introduction

L et me be the first to congratulate you on making an investment in YOU! Not just because belly fat is dangerously unhealthy, but because you will have slimmer, sexier abs if you apply the six methods in this book. You may even get results with just one or two of the methods, or maybe four or five will be needed. It depends upon what's going on in your body.

There are six strategies for losing belly fat without exercise discussed in this book. You will lose belly fat and see a decrease in your waistline while watching your overall health and happiness levels increase to a level you never thought possible.

Right now, I want you to put a tape measure around your waistline because this is the last day you will struggle with belly fat. Measure your results so you can track the inches melting away. Don't forget to e-mail me and let me know how much belly fat you've lost after thirty days.

In "Chapter 1: Remove 7 Fat-Belly Foods," I teach you to remove seven surprising fat-belly foods and to add more of the flat-belly foods. By eating the seven flat-belly foods, you can actually burn belly fat. I also share five guidelines on how to combine foods to help you get the best results. You will also get a seven-day meal plan and recipes for breakfast, lunch, dinner, and snacks to get you started right way.

In "Chapter 2: Discover the 5 Belly-Fat-Blasting Supplements," I discuss the five supplements that will help you burn belly fat. These are not weight-loss pills or pills that suppress your appetite. These are natural supplements that help your own body naturally burn more fat. I will help you cut through the chatter and tell you which ones really work. Here's the trick about supplements: start with just one supplement, maybe two at most, for thirty days. If it's going to work, you will begin noticing its effects after thirty days. This will give it enough time to build up in your system and for you to see if the supplement is going to be effective for you.

In "Chapter 3: Clean the Gut, Lose the Gut," I teach you the two best detox methods that help you lose belly fat. In my bestseller *Lose Weight Without Dieting or Working Out*, I discuss ten different detox methods. Of these, there are two that will specifically help shrink belly fat and bloating. I will explain how to do them, recommend specific products, and tell you where to get them so you can get the best results.

In "Chapter 4: Correct the #1 Hormonal Imbalance That Causes Belly Fat," I will teach you about a condition that often causes belly fat. It doesn't matter what you eat or how much you work out, if you have this hormonal imbalance, you have to correct it in order to get a flat stomach. I will help you figure out if you have this condition and tell you how to correct it.

In "Chapter 5: Avoid 2 Surprising Habits that Cause Belly Fat," I will discuss two bad habits that most of us have picked up with our busy, hectic lives that result in excess belly fat. These are lifestyle changes that can really make a big difference in getting rid of belly fat.

In "Chapter 6: Remove 1 Common Food Allergen That Causes Bloating," you will learn about this common food item that might be contributing to your belly fat and bloating!

The three appendices include frequently asked questions, a seven-day meal plan, and more than fifty recipes that help you get rid of fat, especially stubborn belly fat. The recipes offer variety and make it so much easier to eat delicious meals that burn fat!

One quick note: Throughout this book, when I say "burn fat" I always mean "burn belly fat," but I will often just say "burn fat" to shorten the phrase.

Are you ready to make this commitment to getting a slimmer, sexier waistline? Are you ready to get rid of dangerous belly fat so you can live longer? Are you ready to get that beach body?

Know that this will take resolve, discipline, and the ability to overcome short-term temptation, but those temptations will diminish significantly after the first few weeks. I know how much courage it takes to begin a new life and a new journey to lose weight. I support you and encourage you in your efforts!

CHAPTER ONE

Remove 7 Fat-Belly Foods

There are certain foods that can help your body burn fat, and there are certain foods that make the body store belly fat. In this chapter, I will teach you about the seven surprising fat-belly foods that you will want to eliminate from your diet and the seven flat-belly foods you will want to add to it. I will also share five guidelines on how to combine foods to help you get the best results. (Appendix B provides a seven-day meal plan and recipes for breakfast, lunch, dinner, and snacks to get you started right way.)

When we discuss the seven fat-belly foods that you need to remove from your diet, I don't want you to get too discouraged. It can be really sad to hear the list of foods that cause a fat belly. But there are plenty of other tasty options that can help you burn belly fat.

To get the best results, commit to at least thirty days of removing and adding the foods listed in this chapter. Once you reach your goal and eliminate excess belly fat, having the fat-belly foods on occasion won't be too detrimental. It's when we eat these fat-belly foods on a regular basis that we end up with the persistent belly fat.

THE 7 FAT-BELLY FOODS

As I said earlier, there are certain foods that can help your body burn fat, and there are certain foods that make the body store belly fat. In many cases, the body begins storing fat in as little as two hours after you eat one of these fat-belly foods. If you are serious about getting rid of belly fat, you must remove these seven foods (or as many as possible) from your diet. If you do not remove them, you can expect to have a fat belly for life.

White Sugar

White refined sugar is found in cakes, pies, fruit juices, candy, and so many other things that we crave every day. Many people are addicted to white sugar and don't even know it. I believe this addiction is the main reason people get belly fat. Many people don't think they eat a lot of sugar because they don't eat a lot of sweets like cookies or candy, but the problem is that sugar is hidden in many foods, including bread, muffins, and even dried fruit. I believe sugar is toxic. It has no nutritional value, it's highly addictive, and it makes you sick and fat.

Are you having a panic attack right now just thinking about giving up sugar? You have to look at kicking the sugar habit as though you are ending an addiction. The key is to understand where your sugar is coming from and then find alternatives to eating so much sugar in your foods.

Sugar is measured in grams, and 4 grams of sugar equals one teaspoon. So if your soda has 40 grams of sugar, that's about 10 teaspoons of sugar in just one soda. You can see how so many people end up ingesting so much sugar every day. I used to think I was eating a healthy breakfast by eating oatmeal. However, it wasn't regular oatmeal but the sweetened, flavored, instant oatmeal, like apple-cinnamon oatmeal, and it had about 20 grams of sugar per serving (5 teaspoons!), which is way too much.

As a guideline, the best way to minimize the amount of sugar in your diet is to choose foods that have 5 grams or less per serving. When the drink or food item has 5 grams or less of sugar per serving size, the body doesn't overreact to the sugar. This means your pancreas will not have to release too much insulin. (It's excess insulin that causes belly fat in the body.)

To sweeten foods, it is always better to use stevia or some equivalent herbal sweetener rather than sugar. Stevia is a natural sweetener made from a plant native to South America and Central America. Other countries have been using stevia as a sugar substitute for several decades because it is virtually calorie-free and does not affect blood glucose, which makes it a great natural alternative to sugar and artificial sweeteners.

Sugar will cause belly fat and make you feel irritable, moody, and tired. It can cause numerous health problems, so commit to breaking your sugar addiction today!

Refined Carbohydrates

Because the fiber in refined carbohydrates has been stripped away, they are digested rapidly, causing insulin spikes, which results in fat storage. The foods to avoid are anything made of white flour, including white bread and white pasta. (Furthermore, white flour is bleached nearly the same way you bleach your clothing. When you eat white flour, you're eating some of those bleaching agents, which increases the toxic overload in the body.)

3

Other examples of refined carbs to avoid are bagels, biscuits, donuts, croutons, pancakes, and waffles.

When reading a list of ingredients on a label, don't let the words "wheat flour" or "enriched wheat flour" fool you. It is essentially the same as white flour. You want to look for the label to explicitly say "whole wheat" or "whole grain" when you are buying pastas, breads, and snacks for healthier alternatives. One healthy, whole wheat/whole grain bread alternative is Ezekiel 4:9 brand breads.

So understand what refined carbs are and then avoid them.

White Salt

Sodium, commonly referred to simply as "salt," is another major factor in excess belly fat. Simply put, excess salt causes water retention and bloating. You're going to want to avoid the salt shaker and salt-based seasonings. Better alternatives are sea salt, black pepper, or cayenne pepper, which actually boost your metabolism.

So why does salt cause bloating and heaviness in our belly? Well, water is attracted to sodium, so when you take in high amounts of salt, you retain more fluid—which causes that heavy, puffy appearance and that extra water weight. Foods high in sodium include salty foods like peanuts, French fries, potato chips, and pickles. Look at nutritional labels before you buy any processed foods. Most of us need only 500 to 1,000 milligrams of sodium per day, but too many of us are consuming about six times that much, resulting in large amounts of excess belly fat and bloating.

When you slip up by eating too much of salty foods, drink large amounts of water to flush it out.

Artificial Sweeteners

You know them as those little yellow, pink, and blue packages that are generally marketed as "sugar substitutes." Most people don't realize that even though artificial sweeteners generally have zero calories, they can still contribute to fat gain. These artificial sweeteners increase appetite by sending false signals to the brain that sweet food is on the way. The brain subsequently becomes confused when sweet food never arrives, and so it never gives the signal that you are satisfied. This causes you to crave sugar throughout the day and develop a sweet tooth, sometimes causing you to eat more sugar. Yes, artificial sweeteners can cause you to crave sugar!

Let's look at aspartame, in particular. One study done a few years ago showed that the two main ingredients in aspartame—phenylalanine and aspartic acid—stimulate the release of insulin and leptin, hormones that instruct our bodies to store fat.

The best choice for a calorie-free sweetener is stevia, an herb that grows naturally in parts of Paraguay and Brazil and is now widely available in the United States. You don't need much of it—it's about thirty times sweeter than sugar. Yet it does not raise blood sugar levels or cause rapid-onset cravings the way simple sugars do. A study published in the Journal of Ethno-Pharmacology found that stevia dilates the blood vessels and helps to prevent high blood pressure. It also helps to regulate the digestive system, encourages the growth of friendly bacteria, and helps detoxify the body and excrete more urine naturally.

Trans Fats (Fried Foods)

One of my favorite foods to eat has been my Uncle Spencer's fried fish. It is simply the best. However, I've had to cut back significantly because of the dangers of fried foods. Most fried foods are cooked with partially hydrogenated oils, which contain trans fats. Fried foods become saturated with the hydrogenated oils we use to cook them, and these fat-filled oils cause belly fat. And even worse, you definitely don't want to reuse the oils in which you fry food. Some fast food restaurants do this. Just reusing the cooking oil one time will increase the risk of heart disease.

Some of the foods high in trans fats that can cause belly fat are margarine, commercial baked goods, French fries, onion rings, fried chicken, corn dogs, and funnel cakes, just to name a few.

Just say no to trans fats/fried foods! As an alternative, baked, broiled, or grilled chicken or fish can be just as tasty as their fried versions.

Eating trans fats is like eating plastic and it is very bad for one's health. Trans fats disrupt metabolism, cause weight gain, and increase the risk of diabetes, heart disease, inflammation, and cancer. One Harvard study found that getting just 3 percent of daily calories from trans fats (about 7 to 8 grams of trans fat) increases your risk of heart disease by 50 percent. And given that the average person has about 4 to 10 grams of trans fats in his or her diet each day, it is no wonder heart disease is such a major killer in modern times.

The good news is that the FDA regulates trans fats, and

food manufacturers now have to list how much trans fat is in each serving when in excess of 0.5 grams. So it's now easier to find out how much trans fats are in your foods.

Saturated Fats

Just saying "saturated fats" sounds fat, doesn't it? You will want to minimize foods that are high in saturated fat, as these can lead specifically to belly fat. Saturated fats are found in many common meats, especially red meat, and in whole-fat dairy products like milk and cheese.

The meats to avoid are lamb, poultry, veal, pork, and some cuts of beef. Look for the label to say "lean or extra lean" or choice, select, London broil, or chuck. The worst choices are red meats that say "prime"—they are flavorful but fatty.

Other meat products high in saturated fats are jerky, sausage, and bacon. A better alternative is turkey bacon or turkey sausage.

Whole-fat dairy foods like milk, cream, cheese, and butter are high in saturated fat and can cause belly fat. Cream-based sauces, such as Alfredo, are among the worst.

Let me digress about cow's milk for a second. There are many issues with cow's milk, which is why I encourage almond milk, soymilk, and non-dairy cheeses. I explain that the same way breast milk is made for infant babies, cow's milk is made for infant cows and is difficult for many people to digest. It can lead to inflammation, bloating, and indigestion. Try vegan or non-dairy milk, such as almond, soy, or hemp milk, and non-dairy cheeses.

Eating a lot of saturated fat not only increases belly fat, it also increases cholesterol in the blood and leads to heart attack or stroke. Consumption of these fats should be limited or avoided altogether if possible.

Sodas and Fruit Juices

Let me be as direct as possible regarding this one: sodas and store-bought fruit juices are high in white sugar and/or high-fructose corn syrup and thus cause belly fat. If you are still drinking regular sodas and fruit juices, then just removing those will make a huge difference in getting rid of belly fat!

As a first step, begin substituting diet soda for regular soda. Then gradually decrease the number of diet sodas you drink as well. Although diet sodas are better than regular sodas because they have no sugar, diet sodas still cause some health and weight issues. Diet sodas have been found to make you crave sugar and fattening foods because of the artificial sweeteners in them. Don't replace them with store-bought juices because those contain a lot of sugar and additives that cause weight gain.

A great alternative is green tea (hot or cold), which is a fat burner and helps you lose more weight while still allowing you to get your caffeine fix for the day. You could also try plain water. If that does not sound appealing, try adding a bit of fresh lemon to flavor it.

So, sodas/diet sodas/fruit juices all cause belly fat! Gradually ease off of them. I used to drink three diet sodas a day, now, thankfully, I drink about one to two diet sodas per week. Don't be too hard on yourself. Start to make better food choices one day at a time. It's about progress not perfection!

7 FLAT-BELLY FOODS

The following seven flat-belly foods help you burn fat in two ways: by speeding up your metabolism, reducing insulin levels, and by increasing muscle mass (muscle cells burn more calories than fat). Your goal is to add more of these 7 flat-belly foods into your diet to help burn belly fat.

Lean Fish, Chicken, and Turkey

Lean fish, chicken, and turkey are all good sources of lean protein. The more protein you eat, the harder your body has to work to digest it, resulting in more calories burned during the eating process. The healthiest lean proteins are fish (particularly wild salmon), chicken, and turkey. Avoid the skin on chicken and turkey, as that is where all the saturated fat is found. And of course, we're not going to fry the fish, chicken, or turkey because of the fatty oils (trans fats), but rather bake, broil, grill, or lightly sauté them.

Vegetables

The biggest advantage to eating veggies, particularly the green leafy veggies, is that you can eat them in abundance and still lose weight. The best veggies to eat to burn belly fat are spinach, broccoli, asparagus, kale, collards, turnip greens, mustard greens, beet greens, wheatgrass, carrots, eggplant, celery, peppers, cabbage, cauliflower, Brussels sprouts, and radishes. Try a veggie stir-fry in olive oil with a little cayenne pepper to make a delicious fat-burning meal.

Nuts and Seeds

Nuts and seeds are healthy fats that raise the body's

metabolism and help you burn fat. Nuts and seeds are a great healthy snack option. However, a word of caution: If you want to lose belly fat, or any fat on your body, you should limit your intake of nuts and seeds to one serving (one ounce) per day because they are so calorie-rich; they are a healthy fat, but a fat nonetheless. As long as you don't overeat nuts and seeds, and preferably eat them raw, they promote weight loss and appetite suppression, not weight gain.

So how many nuts make up an ounce? Think "a handful"—what you can hold in your palm. As a tip, I tell my clients to fill up an empty Altoids box with nuts or seeds so you can travel with your handy snack at all times. You don't want to sit in front of the TV watching and eat an entire bag of nuts. Healthy eating means we don't eat out of boredom or for recreation. You want to be disciplined about how you eat and snack!

Berries

Berries are loaded with antioxidants and keep your metabolism going strong. Eat them fresh or frozen. Try blueberries, blackberries, raspberries, and strawberries. In the summer months, they are just marvelous to eat because of how sweet they are. They are a great healthy snack, or you can add them to a protein shake in the morning to replace a heavy breakfast or have them as a snack later in the day.

If fresh berries are unavailable or too expensive, buy frozen ones, puree them in a blender, and drink them as a fruit shake. Easy and delicious!

Green Tea

Studies have shown that green tea is one of the best

metabolism boosters you can drink. Green tea also slows the aging process—it's twenty times more effective in slowing the aging process than vitamin E because of its strong antioxidant capacity, according to some research. There are many wonderful benefits of drinking green tea, but as far as weight loss goes, it simply helps the body burn fat faster and more efficiently. If you've read any of my other books, you know that green tea is one of my most highly recommended beverages to drink to burn fat.

My favorite brand is Wu-long Premium Chinese Slimming Tea.

Cayenne Pepper

Cayenne pepper is known as a fat burner because it fires up your metabolism. It heats up the body, and the body burns calories when it tries to cool itself down. So spice it up for sure! It's so effective, some people actually buy cayenne pepper capsules to burn fat.

Protein Shakes

Protein shakes will help you build muscle, and the more muscle you have, the more calories you burn each day. Protein will also help stabilize blood sugar levels and prevents insulin spikes that result in fat storage.

There are several different types of protein powders available. Whey protein is popular. It is a complete high-quality protein that speeds up metabolism. But it comes from cow's milk, so if you are allergic to dairy, whey protein will cause gas, bloating, and indigestion. My favorite alternatives are rice, soy, and hemp protein powders. If you are a vegetarian, you can use rice protein or a plant-based protein powder to accomplish the same thing.

5 PRINCIPLES ON EATING
TO LOSE BELLY FAT

There are five ways you can eat and combine foods in order to help your body burn belly fat.

Principle 1: Eat Clean Foods

Clean foods are primarily natural, whole, raw, or organic—foods that the body can effectively digest and use for energy without leaving excess waste or toxins in the body. Excess waste in the body ends up in the colon. Where is the colon? In the belly area. We want to get rid of waste in the gut that's making the belly bigger.

Buy organic whenever possible. Organic foods don't have chemical preservatives, food additives, hormones, pesticides, and antibiotics. Fresh organic foods are far less toxic than highly processed and packaged foods and leave less residue and waste in the body. If you can't afford organic fruits and vegetables, wash off the pesticides and waxes as best you can. Waxes are pretty difficult to remove; in fact, they usually can't be removed by simply washing them. You need to purchase special cleansers from health food stores. Be sure to rinse the produce after you scrub off the wax. You can also reduce the toxic content of fruits and vegetables by soaking and scrubbing them in a tub of 10 percent white vinegar and then washing them off with water.

Principle #2: Eat Protein with Every Meal

Eat protein with every meal, and eat it first before the carbohydrates or fats. You can also eat protein by itself. Eating protein does not cause insulin spikes, so it prevents that extra fat from being stored in the body. Protein sources include lean meats (fish, chicken, turkey), eggs, and beans.

Principle #3: Always Balance Carbohydrates with Protein

Whenever you eat a carbohydrate, eat some protein along with it. Examples of some healthy carbohydrates include fruit, vegetables, whole grains, beans, nuts, and seeds. As a general guideline, the protein should be about half the amount of the carbohydrates. For example, if you have 30 grams of carbohydrates, then eat about 15 grams of protein along with it to prevent insulin spikes that cause excess fat to be stored in the body. You can use food labels to determine how much carbs and protein are in food.

Principle #4: Limit Your Intake of Red Meat to Two to Three Times per Week

Most red meat contains a lot of saturated fat, so try to limit your intake to two or three times a week. I told you earlier how to pick "lean red meat" when you're grocery shopping, but until you really understand how to do that, it's best to just limit the amount of red meat to just two, max three times per week. Instead, eat more lean protein from fish, chicken, and other sources, such as eggs, brown rice, beans, and nuts, which contain good essential fats.

Principle #5: Eat Every 3 to 4 Hours

A lot of people diet by eating only once or twice a day, but this is a big mistake. Eating so infrequently significantly slows metabolism and makes it harder for the body to burn belly fat. To burn fat, you should try to eat every three to four hours and think in terms of three meals and two healthy snacks per day. So this is good news! It is important to eat more frequently to burn belly fat!

Now why is that? Every time you eat, you have to burn calories to digest your food. Eating increases your metabolic rate, allowing you to burn fat all day. When you eat only once or twice a day, your body gets a signal telling it that it is food-deprived, causing the body to respond by slowing the metabolic rate and holding on to existing fat reserves to prepare for food scarcity.

To get the best results, commit to at least thirty days of removing and adding the foods listed in this chapter. Once you reach your goal and eliminate excess belly fat, having the occasional fat-belly food won't be too detrimental. It's eating them on a regular basis that causes persistent belly fat.

If you need help with food choices and recipes, refer to the Seven-Day Meal Plan and the 50 Lose-the-Belly Recipes provided in the appendices at the back of this book.

CHAPTER TWO

Discover the 5 Belly-Fat-Blasting Supplements

There are five supplements that I consider best for helping to burn belly fat. These are not weight-loss pills or pills that suppress appetite. These are natural supplements that help your body burn more fat naturally.

Supplements work well for some people but not for others, so you have to experiment a little to get results. If a supplement is going to work for you, it will start working within thirty days. I want to share a few tips on taking supplements. You never want to begin taking three or four supplements at the same time because you won't know which one is working most effectively. Start with only one or two supplements for one month and observe the effect on your body's ability to burn fat. Then, if these don't seem to work, try one or two different supplements.

For dosage, adhere to the instructions on the bottle or follow the advice of a doctor. And, yes, prior to starting any new supplements, be sure to consult with your physician.

The top five belly-fat-blasting supplements are:

- Chromium

- Fish oil
- CLA *(Conjugated Linoleic Acid)*
- Fiber
- Green tea extract

Chromium

My personal favorite supplement for burning fat is chromium—in particular, chromium picolinate. I actually see my belly fat start to come back when I forget to take it for a few weeks. Several studies have shown chromium picolinate to be effective in helping with weight loss, especially in losing belly fat. It is especially good for those who want to lose belly fat and also have diabetes/pre-diabetes or insulin resistance. Now why is this? An increase in belly fat is a side effect of high insulin levels, which lead to insulin resistance, which leads to abdominal fat.

Chromium is a mineral found in the body in trace amounts. Research has shown that chromium supplements in the body help to even out blood-sugar levels while enhancing the body's fat-burning ability. Chromium is also known to be helpful in suppressing cravings for carbs and sugar. For some clients, I recommend it to help them diminish their cravings for sugar and carbs, and it really does a nice job on controlling carbohydrate cravings and improving insulin function in the body.

There are two leading types of chromium supplements: chromium picolinate (my favorite) and chromium polynicotinate. With the chromium polynicotinate supplement, chromium is bound to a form of the B vitamin, niacin. In the picolinate supplement, chromium is combined with the amino acid tryptophan.

There is conflicting information about which type is most effective. Studies have shown that while both types of supplements are safe, chromium polynicotinate is more easily absorbed by the body. There is also more research indicating that chromium polynicotinate promotes more fat loss but preserves muscle mass. I have used both types and, for me, chromium picolinate has been much more effective at fat-burning and weight loss. However, you should do your research and consult with your doctor to choose which type may be best for you.

Fish Oil

Let's look at the fat-burning benefits of taking fish oil and how it causes your body to reduce the amount of body fat it stores. Omega-3 (fish oil) contains three fatty acids (EPA, DHA, and LNA). According to a recent study, these fatty acids aid in the breakdown of fat while also reducing existing fat stores in the body. Omega-3 fatty acids are found in coldwater fish like salmon, mackerel, and sardines. Omega-3s speed up your metabolism and thereby reduce the amount of fat that is stored by the body.

Fish oil will also help you if you have arthritis, joint pain, or heart issues. It helps against inflammation, coronary heart disease, and cancer. Some have found that achy joints start to feel better too—maybe from the lubricating effect of the fish oil.

One of my favorite brands of fish oil is made by Carlson Labs; I like its quality and light lemon and/or orange taste.

CLA (Conjugated Linoleic Acid)

CLA is a natural supplement derived from safflower oil that is used to help the body burn fat without stimulants or other potentially dangerous chemicals. CLA is a healthy fat that helps speed metabolism and does not get stored in the body as fat. CLA decreases fat cells, reduces stored fat, and boosts the body's ability to burn fat.

Researchers have been trying to figure out what causes CLA to keep small fat cells from getting big. The less fat in the cells, the smaller we are and the less fat we'll have in the waist area. For best results, you want to get a quality CLA supplement and take as instructed on the bottle. I can tell you that many take it with the main three meals: breakfast, lunch, and dinner.

Fiber

Research shows that fiber can increase your fat burning by as much as 30 percent. Not only that, a study at Wake Forest Baptist Medical Center showed that eating more fiber can reduce harmful visceral fat (belly fat) and reduce bloating. Fiber is especially helpful if you also have constipation or sluggish bowel movements.

I recommend getting close to 30 grams of fiber per day, as this is the optimum amount for burning fat, preventing disease, and having healthy digestion, including improving bowel regularity. Fiber is a natural appetite suppressant; it curbs your appetite so that you don't overeat throughout the day.

If you don't get 30 grams a day of fiber in your food, there are three options for supplementing your intake.

1. *Acacia-based fiber powder.* Clear, tasteless, zero-calorie acacia fiber can be sprinkled on your food to enhance the fiber content without altering the taste of your meals. Or you can do as I do every day and just

dissolve a scoop in a glass of water and drink it. My favorite brand is called Fiber35 Diet Sprinkle Fiber.

2. *Shakes.* Look for shakes that have at least 10 grams of fiber (from acacia) per serving and avoid shakes that contain artificial sugar substitutes.

3. *Fiber bars.* Look for high-fiber bars that contain oat fiber, acacia fiber, or milled flaxseed and are sweetened with dates, raisins, stevia, or agave syrup.

If you're increasing your fiber intake, it is important to drink plenty of water to avoid constipation. A good rule of thumb is to drink half your body weight in ounces of water daily.

Green Tea Extract

A preliminary animal study showed that drinking green tea daily could prevent up to 76 percent of (belly) fat. There is a growing body of research that shows that green tea can help the body burn belly fat. Green tea is considered a natural fat burner because of the catechins it contains in significant amounts. Additionally, a number of studies have shown that not only does green tea burn belly fat, it also increases your endurance when you are working out. Green tea serves as a glucose regulator, which means it prevents blood-sugar levels from going too high after you have consumed a meal. (Lower blood sugar and insulin levels mean less fat storage in the body.) Green tea is also high in antioxidants, which slow the aging process.

I want to add a side note about the caffeine in green tea. About half the research shows caffeine to be beneficial, and about half suggests it has detrimental effects on the body. I'm with the half that says it can be beneficial and can improve the fat-burning process. Thus, I recommend drinking some caffeinated drinks like green tea in moderation.

Green tea is better than black tea or coffee because its caffeine works in a different way. Green tea makes the body's own energy use more efficient, thereby improving vitality and stamina without your having to experience the ups and downs typically caused by ingesting caffeine. This is due to the large amount of tannins in green tea that ensure that the caffeine is taken to the brain in only small amounts, which harmonizes the energies in the body.

My favorite brand is Wu-long Premium Chinese Slimming Tea; keep in mind that green tea actually reduces fat all over the body, not just the belly. So add green tea to your diet and see how great it helps you look and feel!

So pick one or two of these supplements, add them to your daily regimen, and monitor their effects on your belly fat. Do this for thirty days. Some supplements will work better than others for your unique body.

CHAPTER THREE

Clean the Gut, Lose the Gut

In my book Lose Weight Without Dieting or Working Out, I describe twelve different detox methods that help with weight loss. In this chapter, I will discuss the two that do the most to specifically help you shrink belly fat and reduce bloating.

Now, I'm going to have to really level set everyone to get us all on the same page. Before I give you the two detox methods, I don't want to assume everyone knows what it means to detox the body for weight loss. This is important to understand before I give you the detox methods that help to flatten the belly.

What's Making Us Unhealthy and Overweight?

I often tell the story of how I was coaching a client a while back and she asked me a very poignant question. She said, "Why am I always sick and what's making me fat?" I said to her that is not the question of the day, but the question of the century. Toxins make us fat and they make us sick! And they are the missing piece to the puzzle as to why we can't lose weight and why we feel unhealthy and sick!

We live in a toxic environment. As we get older, we've lived long enough for all the toxins we take in every day to build up in our bodies and create a toxic overload. Major illness (diabetes, high blood pressure, arthritis, asthma) is so commonplace that we don't even pay attention to it. Our grandparents had less stress and ate cleaner food, and a hundred years ago today's big three diseases (cancer, diabetes, and heart disease) were relatively rare. Elderly people didn't need to have a tackle box of pills just to make it through the day.

So it's not just how much you're eating that's causing you to gain weight, it is WHAT you're eating and what your body is exposed to that are causing a toxic overload in your body.

What Are Toxins?

A toxin is any substance that irritates or creates harmful effects in the body. Toxins are everywhere—in our food, of course, but also in our air and water, our skin and hair care products, our carpets and furniture, our cleaning fluids, etc. We are unknowingly filling our bodies with toxins that have burdened our systems.

There are two types of toxins—internal and environmental. Internal toxins are the waste products—like bacteria, fungi, and yeast—in the body that need to be released. Environmental toxins include pollutants, drugs, hormones/birth control pills, prescription medications, household cleaners, food additives, pesticides, and others. The Standard American Diet (SAD) includes a ton of processed foods with low nutritional value and quite a number of different toxins that are considered "safe" by the FDA but which build up over time to have negative effects.

A toxic body is not only dangerously unhealthy but it slows metabolism, decreasing your ability to burn fat by up to 20 percent.

So, How Do Toxins Make Us Fatter?

Detoxification, which is the process of removing toxins from the body, is critical to losing fat because many of the toxins the body holds onto are stored in fat cells. When the body does not know what to do with all the toxins we take in every day, it stores them as fat cells. The more toxins we take in, the more fat cells we have in our body. Since fat cells don't break down very easily, they literally weigh down the body and make it bigger.

The following symptoms indicate the presence of excess toxins in the body: bloating, constipation, indigestion, low energy, fatigue/brain fog, depression, weight gain, chronic pain, infections, allergies, headaches, and gut/digestion problems.

DETERMINING WHETHER YOU HAVE EXCESS TOXINS IN YOUR BODY

Take this quiz to determine whether you have toxic overload in your body that is leading to extra fat being stored in your body.

Are Excess Toxins Causing Your Weight Gain? Self-Assessment Quiz!

If you are dealing with fatigue, weight gain, chronic disease, an inability to focus, or accelerated aging, you will want to take this quiz to determine if toxic overload in your body is the underlying cause. Take this quiz and score your results to gain a sense of how much toxic burden you're carrying in your body.

Read each question and give yourself one point for every yes answer.

- ☐ Do you crave sweets, bread, pasta, white rice, and/or potatoes?

- ☐ Do you eat processed foods (TV dinners, lunch-meats, canned foods) or fast foods at least three times a week?

- ☐ Do you drink caffeinated beverages like coffee and tea more than three times daily?

- ☐ Do you drink diets sodas or use artificial sweeteners at least once a day?

- ☐ Do you sleep less than eight hours per day?

- ☐ Do you drink less than 64 ounces of good, clean water daily?

- ☐ Are you very sensitive to smoke, chemicals, or fumes in the environment?

- ☐ Have you ever taken antibiotics, antidepressants, or other medications?

- ☐ Have you ever taken birth control pills or other estrogens, such as hormone replacement therapy?

- ☐ Do you have frequent yeast infections?

- ☐ Do you have "silver" dental fillings?

- ☐ Do you use commercial household cleaners, cosmetics, or deodorants?

- ☐ Do you eat non-organic vegetables, fruits, or meat?

- ☐ Have you ever smoked or been exposed to secondhand smoke?

- ☐ Are you overweight or do you have cellulite fat deposits?

- ☐ Does your occupation expose you to environmental toxins?

- ☐ Do you live in a major metropolitan area or near a big airport?

- ☐ Do you feel tired, fatigued, or sluggish throughout the day?

- ☐ Do you have difficulty concentrating or focusing?

- ☐ Do you suffer bloating, indigestion, or frequent gas after eating?

- ☐ Do you get more than two colds or the flu per year?

- ☐ Do you have reoccurring congestion, sinus issues, or postnasal drip?

- ☐ Do you sometimes notice you have bad breath, a coated tongue, or strong-smelling urine?

- ☐ Do you have puffy eyes or dark circles under your eyes?

- ☐ Are you often sad or depressed?

- ☐ Do you often feel anxious, antsy, or stressed?

- ☐ Do you have acne, breakouts, rashes, or hives?

- ☐ Do you have less than one bowel movement per day and/or get constipated occasionally?

- ☐ Do you have insomnia or trouble getting restful sleep?

☐ Do you get blurred vision or itchy, burning eyes?

Results

The higher your score, the greater the potential toxic burden you may be carrying and the more you may benefit from a detoxification and cleansing program.

- *If you scored 20 or higher:* You will significantly benefit from detoxifying your body, which could lead to weight loss and improved health and vitality. It is strongly recommended that you look into different ways to detoxify the body.

- *If you scored between 5 and 19:* You will likely benefit from a detoxification program for improved health and vitality.

- *If you scored below 5:* You might actually be free of toxic overload in the body and are living a very healthy, toxin-free life. Good for you!

Although our bodies have the ability to eliminate toxins, it's when the body gets overloaded with toxins that they start to contribute to weight gain and health issues. Here's why: When the body is overwhelmed with the toxins we take in every day, it stores them in fat cells. Fat cells don't get broken down very easily, so they literally weigh down the body and make it bigger. As toxins accumulate, we begin to experience health problems like allergies, migraines, major diseases, and fatigue/low energy.

DETOXIFICATION 101: THE BASICS

So what is detoxification? Detoxification is a total-body cleansing process for all of the body's detoxification organs and systems. It is the process of cleansing and reducing the toxic overload that resides in the body. A few words that are interchangeable: "detoxification," "cleansing," and "detox."

Many people falsely think of the word "cleanse" as a one-time fast, or colon-cleanse, that is done for a few days every few years. This is detoxification in a very narrow sense. Although the colon is one of the many detoxification channels for elimination, total body cleansing goes far beyond colon cleansing. It involves cleansing all of the organs involved in natural detoxification in the body, including the liver, kidneys, skin, etc.

Just as you wouldn't wait a year to clean your house, you shouldn't wait a year to "cleanse" your inner body. Regular cleansing ensures that you are constantly eliminating toxins and getting rid of waste and sludge. If you wait too long to cleanse the body, toxins get deeper into the body, making you look and feel tired and old, eventually leading to disease and weight gain.

Thus, we have to think of cleansing as a regular, ongoing activity we do to reach our highest potential for optimum health and wellness.

Detoxing differs from dieting in that its primary goal is to cleanse the entire body. However, one of the natural outcomes of detoxing is that excess weight melts away. As we eliminate toxins from the fat cells, the fat cells shrink and we get smaller.

Helping the body cleanse is not unnatural nor is it a one-time thing. I have clients, friends, and doctors who regularly detoxify the body for optimum health.

Benefits of detoxifying the body:

- Weight loss and the realization that you can enjoy a lighter style of eating.
- Improved digestion, including less acid reflux, constipation, gas, bloating.
- Fewer allergic or reactive responses to foods.
- Less throat and lung congestion.
- More energy.
- Better nutrient absorption, leading to overall improved health.
- Sense of satisfaction, greater vitality, and a desire to choose better foods that help the body feel alive and energetic.
- A deeper understanding of how to take care of yourself and achieve optimum health.

When you begin detoxifying the body, you may notice a change for the better in your health and energy levels within a few days; however, for others, it may take a few months. Everyone's toxic overload is different, and many factors come into play, such as your health status, weight, metabolism, age, and genetics. But you will be rewarded with better health in the end.

DETOX METHOD #1: COLON CLEANSING

Let's talk about the first detox method that will reduce belly fat and bloating: the colon. The colon's function is to remove waste from the body. When the colon doesn't function properly, toxic waste accumulates in the digestive tract. When you eat a poor diet without essential nutrients, fecal matter residue remains on the intestinal walls, creating a plaque-like substance that is not at all good for health. This is disgusting, I know, but it has been said that the average healthy person has five to ten pounds of dried fecal matter present in the colon. The potbelly many people are unable to lose despite regular exercise might actually be due to accumulated waste in the colon. It may be possible to lose up to ten pounds of waste from the colon/abdominal area by simply cleansing the colon. Many people with "potbellies" may actually have several pounds of old, hardened fecal matter lodged within their colons. As a result, the process will actually cause you to experience some immediate weight loss.

One way to cleanse the colon is to use colon-cleansing herbs. They come in the form of powdered or capsule supplements. Their purpose is to force the colon to expel its contents. Colon cleansing not only helps remove the junk from intestinal walls, it also allows waste to pass through more freely, which helps reduce constipation and bloating.

Different colon-cleansing herbs perform different actions. Some work to help you eliminate fecal matter and prevent toxic buildup; others kill harmful bacteria and parasites; others soften the stool, add bulk, and improve the function of colon muscles to promote healthy and regular bowel movements. You want to get one that really eliminates waste/fecal matter and kills harmful bacteria and parasites. When you see what comes out in your stool, you will be amazed . . . and possibly disgusted.

Here are three options for colon-cleansing herbs. I have no relationship with these companies, as they don't pay me to endorse their products. These are the products my clients and I have used and know to be very effective.

- *Top-tier:* This is a thirty-day cleanse. It cleanses all the detox organs—colon, liver, kidneys, skin. If you've never done any colon cleansing, this is a good one to plan on doing in the spring or whenever you have time to commit to thirty days. My favorite thirty-day cleanse is a product by Blessed Herbs.

- *Mid-tier:* This ten-day cleanse involves taking herbs/supplements and liquid powder drinks in the morning and at night. It is very effective. My favorite product is Colonix by DrNatura.

- *Low-tier:* This is called low-tier only because of its lower price, as it is still incredibly effective. You can get started and get immediate results, even overnight. I like two products in particular: Triphala and a magnesium-oxide supplement called Mag07. Triphala gently cleanses the digestive tract and rids the body of toxins. My favorite is one made by Planetary Herbals. Mag07 is a very powerful and effective colon cleanser that releases oxygen over twelve hours or more throughout the entire digestive system. The magnesium acts as a vehicle to transport the oxygen throughout the body and has the gentle effect of loosening toxins and acidic waste and transporting them out of the body. Mag07 is a product that is truly a personal favorite of mine! You just take three to five tablets at bedtime, along with two Triphala tablets. You will have a heavy release each morning. Do this for seven days and you will get a very good digestive cleanse.

Colonics

Another option for colon cleansing is colon hydrotherapy, or colonics, a procedure used to remove waste and impacted fecal matter from the colon. Colonics works while you lie on a table; a colonics therapist uses a machine or gravity-driven pump to slowly flush up to twenty gallons of water through a tube inserted into the rectum. The therapists may use a variety of water pressures and temperatures. The procedure takes forty-five minutes to an hour.

It is a common misconception that doing colonics will cause the body to get rid of all the good bacteria along with the bad. If you decide to do a colonic, it will rinse out the good bacteria, the probiotics, in your colon—but just temporarily. After you flush out everything, your body will replace the good bacteria within twenty-four hours unless you are extremely unhealthy or weak. However, you should always take a probiotic supplement after a colonic to aid in this replenishment of the good bacteria right away. A good colon therapist will always provide you with probiotics at the end of your colonics session.

If you choose to research colonics and decide to include them as part of your detoxification process, you probably want to go at least once a week for up to six weeks, particularly when you first begin aggressively detoxifying the body. That is because you are drawing out toxins in the body, and if they are not eliminated quickly, they can cause detox symptoms that become uncomfortable.

One rule of thumb as to whether to do a colonic is determined by how frequent your bowel movements are. If your body is managing the toxins and waste well through normal daily bowel movements (one to two per day), then you probably don't need to have a colonic. If your bowel movements are less frequent than once a day, it may be a good idea to do a colonic to get your bowels moving more frequently.

DETOX METHOD #2: LIVER CLEANSE

The liver (also known as the fat-burning organ) is responsible for breaking down fats and eliminating toxins. When the liver is overloaded with toxins, it has a difficult time eliminating them, so it begins to store the toxins in fat cells. When your liver functions efficiently, it is much easier to lose weight because the liver will eliminate toxins and metabolize fats rather than store excess fat in the body.

Trying to lose weight without getting rid of the toxins guarantees you will gain it right back. You might eat less and exercise in an attempt to lose fat, but if you do not also get rid of the toxins, they get reabsorbed into the body and create more fat cells.

If you have body fat accumulation, especially around the waist and midsection, it suggests that your liver may not be functioning properly or as efficiently as it could. That's what is called a "sluggish liver" or "fatty liver." In fact, over 90 million Americans are believed to have fatty livers. It means the liver may have stopped processing fat and stores it right around the waistline. Thus, detoxifying the liver leads to a slimmer waistline.

Some people will argue that the liver is fully capable of processing toxins. True, it is, until it gets overloaded, which slows its ability to metabolize and burn fats, and then it starts storing fats in the body.

Things that make it difficult for the liver to eliminate toxins include residue of herbicides/pesticides in foods, artificial sweeteners, over-the-counter pain relievers, excess alcohol, and medications. We often hear on the TV ads for medications that people should not use them if they are being treated for liver problems. That is because the liver has to be very healthy to be able to process these medicines.

Let's take a look at the routines in just one day of a person's life that may cause extra stress on the liver. Let's say this person starts the day by taking medicine for high blood pressure. Then she has a headache around noon, so she pops a painkiller. She eats at a fast food restaurant for lunch and ingests processed foods. She doesn't have a bowel movement all day. After work, she has three drinks at happy hour. All of these things put extra stress on the liver, making it more difficult to eliminate toxins.

The following symptoms are signs of a sluggish liver:
- Poor skin tone or flushed facial appearance
- Discoloration of the eyes
- Dark circles
- Yellow-coated tongue
- Acne or breakouts around the nose, cheeks, and chin
- Bitter taste in the mouth
- Headaches
- Moodiness and irritability

- Excessive sweating
- Excessive facial blood vessels
- Red palms and soles, which may also be itchy and inflamed

So how do you keep the liver healthy? By doing a liver cleanse. One easy cleanse can be done by taking herbs/supplements, such as milk thistle, dandelion root, and burdock. These herbs are all-natural and are very effective at liver detoxification. You'll find that many products on the market combine these herbs into one supplement so that you can achieve the best results. Be sure to use only products that are all-natural and gentle on the body. My favorite two liver cleansing supplements are Liver Rescue by Healthforce and Livatone Plus by Dr. Sandra Cabot.

An inexpensive way to cleanse the liver is to drink two tablespoons of apple cider vinegar in eight ounces of water every morning and night. Do this for two to three weeks or continue until your sluggish liver symptoms have improved. My favorite brand is Bragg Apple Cider Vinegar.

It's also a good idea to eat and drink detoxifying foods like green tea or liver-loving foods such as green leafy vegetables, including mustard greens, kale, spinach, or to eat more citrus fruits like oranges, lemons, and limes. These foods detoxify the body and keep the liver clean.

Completing a liver cleanse can be a positive and rejuvenating experience and yield numerous health benefits. As you improve liver health, you increase your body's ability to detoxify itself, improve its fat-burning capabilities, and achieve optimum health.

Detoxing through colon cleansing and liver cleansing will help flatten the belly and reduce bloating and water weight as well as improve your health and energy!

CHAPTER FOUR

Correct the #1 Hormonal Imbalance That Causes Belly Fat

I don't care what you eat or if you work out, if you have this hormonal imbalance, you have to correct it in order to get a flat stomach. In this chapter, I will help you figure out if you have this hormonal imbalance and how to correct it.

Are you over thirty-five and beginning to notice a few extra pounds around your waist and belly area? You may not have changed your eating habits or exercise routine but may still be unable to maintain your weight. You should be happy to know that you are definitely not alone. Over 90 percent of women gain weight between the ages of thirty-five and fifty-five—about fifteen to twenty pounds to be exact—but this is normal and happens to most of us. However, it doesn't mean we have to keep it! It's not just that we gain weight, it's also how the weight tends to be distributed around the waistline, belly, thighs, hips, and butt area that makes the body appear more round and less curvy, often making us pear-shaped or apple-shaped.

Both men and woman over the age of thirty-five tend to

gain weight due to fluctuating hormones. The good news is that you can achieve a better hormone balance that gets rid of the extra fat around the stomach, hips, and thighs. You do not have to accept that extra belly bulge as you age, and yes, you can lose that extra fat!

Now let me give you a few facts about hormonal decline over age thirty-five. Sorry if this sounds like a medical class, but there are a few key concepts that are important to understand. There are three key sex hormones that decline as you age: estrogen, progesterone, and testosterone.

Estrogen

Estrogen is produced by the ovaries, and is what transforms girls into women. It gives us our curves and helps regulate our passage through fertility and menstruation. Both men and women have estrogen, but women have much higher levels.

Progesterone

A woman's body secretes *progesterone* every month after an egg is released. This hormone helps the body burn fat and can help reduce bloating and water weight. The sudden appearance of abdominal fat is a sign that the body's internal hormonal ratio of progesterone to estrogen is unbalanced. So the primary goal is to restore the balance between estrogen and progesterone because when they are properly balanced, these two hormones help the body burn fat, especially belly fat.

Testosterone

Many women are surprised to hear that they actually produce *testosterone*. Men naturally make 50 percent more testosterone than women; however, it is a vital hormone in women also. It helps us maintain our energy level, muscle tone, vaginal elasticity, sex drive, and overall vitality. But when we have too much testosterone, it causes acne and facial hair. Have you seen women with facial hair above the lip and under the chin? They likely have too much testosterone in their system.

As we age, we all experience a decline in hormone levels. But I'm going to teach you how to achieve a better hormonal balance so you can get rid of that stubborn belly fat and other unpleasant symptoms.

WHAT IS ESTROGEN DOMINANCE?

Estrogen dominance is the primary hormonal imbalance that causes excess belly fat. When estrogen levels remain high in the body relative to progesterone, the result is a condition known as estrogen dominance. The primary symptoms of estrogen dominance are weight gain (especially around the waist and abdomen), mood swings, and bloating.

Both men and women can suffer from estrogen dominance. If you gained extra belly fat after you turned thirty-five, estrogen dominance is the likely cause.

I know of estrogen dominance all too well, and every one of these symptoms was very real and very frustrating to me. Additionally, if you are struggling with all over body fat, then you may also want to get tested for low thyroid function, which is another hormonal imbalance that causes steady weight gain throughout the body.

Estrogen dominance also causes increased bloating and

water retention; the extra weight may not be the result of more fat but will still make you look heavier. Estrogen dominance causes your blood sugar to fluctuate, which increases your appetite and slows your metabolism. Women often experience bloating when they are menstruating. When women no longer have periods and are not producing progesterone, the bloating will be a constant problem. Progesterone acts as a natural diuretic. Progesterone also encourages the body to use calories from food for energy; without enough progesterone, the body is compromised in its ability to metabolize calories, and the calories get stored as fat in the body.

Contrary to the popular belief that estrogen is a "female" hormone, men can also be estrogen dominant. One possible cause of estrogen dominance is exposure to environmental estrogens, and men are exposed to the same ones as women. Men who show signs of estrogen dominance are typically over the age of forty and experience weight gain around the middle, hair loss, development of breasts (man boobs), and fatigue.

The "thickening" of women's bodies and the "softening" of men's bodies are often related to excess estrogen. In excess, estrogen promotes the growth of estrogen-sensitive tissues, known as "stubborn fat," because they are highly resistant to fat burning. Even eating less and exercising doesn't help remove the estrogen-sensitive fat. You get caught in a vicious cycle as excess estrogen promotes fat gain; the enlarged estrogen-sensitive fat tissue produces more estrogen within its cells, which then promotes more fat gain, and so on.

Here are some common symptoms of estrogen dominance. Put a check mark next to the symptoms you have; the more symptoms you have, the more likely you are dealing with estrogen dominance:

- Stubborn fat/weight gain around stomach area, hips, thighs
- Water retention/bloating
- Tender breasts
- Low libido
- Problematic PMS/menstrual cramps
- Dry skin/vaginal dryness
- Mood swings or irritability
- Hot flashes/night sweats
- Insomnia
- Brain fog or "fuzzy thinking"
- Irregular periods or heavy or long-lasting periods
- Fatigue
- Depression or low motivation
- Cyclical migraine headaches
- Infertility or frequent miscarriage
- Fibrocystic breasts
- Uterine fibroids
- Endometriosis
- Polycystic ovary syndrome (PCOS)
- Breast cancer

If you have the majority of these symptoms, you may be suffering from estrogen dominance.

WHAT TO DO ABOUT
ESTROGEN DOMINANCE

There are ten things you can do to reduce the symptoms of estrogen dominance, thereby eliminating excess stubborn body and belly fat.

1. *Maintain healthy bowel and liver function.* Regular bowel movements are the best way to keep estrogen moving through and out of the body. You should have one to three bowel movements per day. Yes, I started the list with healthy bowel movements (smile).

2. *Avoid alcohol.* Sorry! How about trying to *minimize* alcohol first? It spurs the production of harmful estrogen. In fact, even one glass of alcohol a day can raise estrogen levels.

3. *Minimize exposure to xenoestrogens.* These are environmental chemicals in pesticides, plastics, some cosmetics, and household cleaning products that can get into your bloodstream and increase estrogen levels. These xenoestrogens act like estrogen in the body.

4. *Eliminate sugar and starch from your diet.* Get sugar out of your diet if you want to lose belly fat. This means candy, cookies, and other sweets, of course, but also all starchy processed foods that cause insulin spikes that result in excess fat in the body.

5. *Eat more fiber.* Fiber from whole grains, fruits, and vegetables help move estrogen out of the body, which helps prevent it from building up and creating a hormonal burden on your system. You can also do

fiber shakes, fiber bars, etc. Try to get 30 grams of fiber per day.

6. *Eat lean proteins.* I often talk about the value of lean protein, but it really helps to offset the symptoms of estrogen dominance by helping you maintain muscle mass, which burns more calories than fat. Good choices of protein are eggs, beans, fish, turkey, or chicken.

7. *Eat more detoxifying foods.* These are foods that cleanse the body, so add plenty of detoxifying foods to your diet, such as broccoli, cauliflower, Brussels sprouts, kale, cabbage, beets, carrots, apples, ginger, onions, and celery. Eat at least five servings of fresh fruits and veggies per day. In particular, dark leafy green veggies, such as spinach, collards, and kale, are ideal. The best fruit choices are those with the brightest and deepest colors, such as oranges, black-berries, and apples.

8. *Look into natural hormone therapy, called bio-identical hormone replacement therapy (BHRT), to restore hormonal balance.* Now if you had the majority of the symptoms we discussed earlier, then you might want to look into this advanced strategy. Bio-identical hormones help you restore a good hormonal balance between estrogen and progesterone. They are hormones derived from plants, usually soybeans or wild yams, through a biochemical process that ensures that the molecular structure is identical to the hormones women make in their own bodies, and they are very natural to the body. In my book *Lose Weight Without Dieting or Working Out*, I provide

a detailed discussion on bio-identical hormones, focusing on where and how to use them. So I don't want to digress too much into that in this book. However, you can work with a doctor and get a hormone panel test to find out if bio-identical hormones can help you restore your hormonal balance.

9. *Look into DIM. Diindolylmethane (DIM) is a natural supplement that helps alleviate the symptoms of estrogen dominance.* It is a phytonutrient, a plant compound similar to those found in cruciferous vegetables, such as broccoli, cabbage, Brussels sprouts, and cauliflower. Since it would be difficult to get enough of these vegetables in the diet daily (it would require eating two pounds of broccoli per day) to properly eliminate the bad estrogen, we can take a nutritional supplement known as DIM to get the adequate amounts to restore hormonal balance and eliminate the symptoms of estrogen dominance. DIM eliminates excess estrogen by shifting the way estrogen is metabolized in the body. DIM allows for more of the "good estrogen" metabolites and elimination of the "bad estrogen" metabolites. Read some of the product reviews on DIM and you'll see that people get great results.

10. *Get moving!* The unpleasant reality is that women begin to naturally lose muscle mass during middle age. Not only are we gaining and storing fat, we're losing lean muscle mass as well. This is a double whammy. You will want to begin some physical activity to help maintain lean muscle mass as you age to boost your metabolism.

When I wrote my book *Lose Weight Without Dieting or Working Out*, I experienced many unpleasant symptoms of estrogen dominance, including acne, bloating, depression, hot flashes, heavy or painful periods, irregular periods, irritability (I'm lucky to still have my family and friends!), loss of muscle mass, mood swings, poor concentration, sleep disturbances, urinary incontinence, and, my least favorite, the unexplained sudden appearance of belly fat. My fat belly was actually alarming due to how healthy my lifestyle and eating habits were at the time.

By following the ten strategies to balance my hormones, I learned one thing: that a healthy woman is hormonally balanced.

If you are frustrated with belly fat, a pear- or apple-shaped body, or bloating and water retention, these strategies may help you melt the fat away.

CHAPTER FIVE

Avoid 2 Surprising Habits that Cause Belly Fat!

There are two surprising habits that cause belly fat— yes, bad habits that we've picked up due to our busy, hectic lives are causing our belly fat!

Habit #1: Too Much Stress

The first bad habit that causes belly fat is having too much STRESS in our lives all the time. This is stress, mess, drama, whatever you want to call it. It's scientifically proven that stress causes belly fat! Now think about how much belly fat you have and then think about how much stress and drama you have in your life. See any correlation? (SMILE)

So how does stress cause belly fat? One word: cortisol!

When you are stressed, your body releases cortisol, and fat caused by stress stores in the belly. Cortisol is also nicknamed the stress hormone. So the short story is that high cortisol levels increase belly fat. Studies have shown that an increase in cortisol increases the fat around the belly, increases your hunger, and leads to more cravings.

When cortisol is released into the bloodstream, you become less sensitive to leptin, the hormone that tells your brain you are full. When this happens, you tend to eat more and begin to crave sugar. That means that your body not only slows down your metabolism when you are stressed out, it actually tells you to consume more food.

Here's how it works: Cortisol is released in larger amounts during times of stress, producing the "fight-or-flight" response. Then the hormone triggers a hunger response in the brain, signaling cells to store as much fat as possible.

To lose belly fat, you are going to need to reduce your cortisol levels, and to do that is going to require some lifestyle changes that reduce stress! You can have your cortisol levels tested with a 24-hour saliva test. This is the most effective way to determine your cortisol levels throughout the day.

Yes, eliminating stress can help you lose belly fat. To reduce the stress in your life, follow these tips:

- *Do a mental detox by avoiding toxic people.* Just as you must clean the toxins out of your body, you also need to clean out the poisonous thoughts and feelings that come from family and friends who cause unnecessary stress and drama in your life. People who belittle you and make you feel unworthy should get very little of your time. These people trigger stress and negative emotions in your life. Sometimes they can just say hello, and your stress level increases because you know at the end of that interaction, you will feel low, hurt, or sad. Take steps to minimize the time you spend with these people.

- *Love yourself and make YOU a priority.* When you have positive feelings about who you are, you send a signal to others that you have value and deserve respect. Loving yourself sends a clear message that you are to be recognized, celebrated, appreciated, and loved. Sometimes our sense of self-worth or self-esteem is shaped by the people in our inner circle. Some of us have family members and friends ruining our self-esteem every day. Even if they are your flesh and blood, try to remove yourself from their presence as much as possible. Self-love is so essential to survival. There is no successful, authentic relationship with others without self-love. We cannot nurture others from a dry well. It is not selfish or self-indulgent. We have to take care of our needs first so we can give to others from our abundance. Please make LOVING YOU a priority!

- *Place "happy photos" at work and in your car (like on the visor).* When you look at them, they will immediately take you to a happy place, causing stress levels to decrease.

- *Make love.* The more we make love, the more endorphins our brains release. These neuro-hormones that are released in the brain act as natural painkillers and help to alleviate anxiety. Sex makes you feel good, unless you're doing it all wrong!

- *Schedule "playtime" with your significant other or children.* Doing fun things like miniature golf, bowling, and seeing a movie can take your mind off your stress.

- *Smile often and laugh a lot.* If you have a favorite comedian, include a CD in your car to listen to as you drive to and from work. Or watch movies that make you laugh out loud. Or listen to music that calms you down or makes you sing along. What is your favorite song that, when you hear it, you just light up . . . play this song often!

- *Get or give a massage.* Deep-pressure massage stimulates nerves that reduce cortisol levels. Research has also shown that those who give massages reduce their own levels of stress hormones. So giving or receiving massages helps tremendously.

- *Get moving.* It is well documented that regular physical activity or exercise helps to alleviate stress and raise your body temperature, which helps the body prepare for sleep. There's strong evidence that moderate exercise like brisk walking activates the "feel good" neurotransmitters dopamine and serotonin, which reduce the symptoms of depression.

- *Do your part to build better relationships.* I once asked someone, "What's the common denominator in all of your failed relationships?" The answer is *you!* If you struggle to build meaningful, loving relationships, try showing more respect and compassion for other people, maybe even more than you feel they deserve. This might seem to hurt you in the short term, but it is a sure investment in the long term.

- *If lack of time stresses you out, learn to master time management.* Time management is an art, and you can learn better time management skills. The best book that I've ever read about time management is called *How to Get Control of Your Time and Your Life* by Alan Lakein. It is definitely worth reading.

- **Take a stress supplement.** When all else fails, try a supplement/herb that will protect against the physical toll stress has on our bodies. A few examples are Dr. Wilson's Super Stress Formula or Adrenal Rebuilder, or Gaia Herbs Adrenal Health. These are a last resort if other suggestions don't work.

I want you to seriously think about how you're going to get some of the stress out of your life. Think of three things or three people who stress you out. Then think about how you can improve these situations.

Don't underestimate the toll stress takes on your health and well-being and certainly on your weight and body shape as well.

Habit #2: Lack of Sleep

Another bad habit that will be essential to change in order to lose belly fat is to get more sleep!

Many Americans are sleep-deprived, and perhaps you are one of them. Here's something you probably don't know: Sleep helps you burn fat! An interesting 2010 study found that dieters who slept 8.5 hours a night lost twice as much fat as those who got 5.5 hours of sleep or less. You mean to tell me that sleep can help you burn twice as much fat? In fact, by the end of the study, the long sleepers were burning an extra 115 calories per day (that's about 10 pounds a year)! Whoa!

Additionally, sleep deprivation tends to lead to food

cravings, particularly for sweet and starchy foods. Researchers have suggested that these sugar cravings stem from the fact that the brain is fueled by glucose (blood sugar). Therefore, when it is sleep-deprived, the brain starts searching for carbs to keep it going. The extra sugar will, of course, cause you to gain weight.

So this is a simple habit to change: Get more sleep! So many Americans are sleep-deprived. However, I can honestly say I am not one of them. I am a huge fan of sleep. In fact, I'm a member of a Facebook fan page called SLEEP! We talk about getting better sleep and just appreciating sleep! But seriously, I get my eight hours of sleep every night, and if I fall short one night, I make up for it over the weekend.

Sleep is the body's way of recharging the system and is the easiest yet most underrated activity to heal the body. Sleep also helps to eliminate puffy red eyes and dark circles. There isn't anything that can compensate for lack of sleep. Lack of sleep causes extra wear and tear on the body, accelerating aging, and pushes the body out of its natural balance and rhythm. Short-changing sleep time or going to bed stressed interferes with the best time for losing those extra pounds. So be sure to relax or meditate before going to sleep. In short, getting enough sleep helps you burn more calories both at night and during the day.

Okay, hopefully, I've convinced you to get more quality sleep. Now the goal is get good, restful sleep. I'm going to give you several tips and the key is to experiment. What works for some might not work as well for others. It's important to find the sleep strategies that work best for you.

Now the first step to improving the quality of your rest is finding out how much sleep you need. How much sleep is enough—7.5, 8, 8.5 hours? Sleep requirements vary slightly from person to person. Most healthy adults need at least eight hours of sleep each night to function at their best. If you are not getting enough sleep, here are a few habits that can help you to do so.

- *Keep a regular sleep schedule.* If you go to bed and get up at the same time each day, you will feel much more refreshed and energized than if you sleep at different times and for a different amount of hours. Consistency is important. My friends laugh at me because I go to sleep by 9:30 p.m. but wake up pretty refreshed around 5:30 a.m. every day! So try to go to bed at the same time every night—whenever you normally get tired, whatever that is for you. Try not to mess up on the weekends when it may be tempting to stay up late.

- *Take naps.* A good nap can make up for lost sleep, and doing that is much better than letting sleep deprivation build up over weeks and months. If you need to make up for a few lost hours, try to sneak in a daytime nap rather than sleeping late. A good nap typically lasts for about ten to thirty minutes. Don't do two hours, as that will really mess up your sleep cycle. And please don't nap at your desk at work!

- *Fight after-dinner sleepiness.* If you find yourself getting sleepy in the evening after you eat, but well before your bedtime, get off the couch and do something mildly stimulating to avoid falling asleep, such as washing the dishes, calling a friend, or getting clothes ready for the next day. If you give in to the drowsiness, you may wake up in the middle of the night, and then you'll have trouble getting back to sleep. No good!

- *Make a "to-do" list just before bedtime.* When we lie down to go to sleep, often our minds are racing like crazy, thinking about all we have to do the next day—pay bills, respond to e-mails, finish chores, etc. If you can't shut off these thoughts, it helps to make a list of everything you need to do the next day. This really works for me. Otherwise, I can make myself crazy thinking about all the stuff I need to do! If you make a list, it will help you put these thoughts aside and relax enough to fall asleep.

- *Establish a bedtime routine.* This can be soaking in a hot bath, meditating, praying, reading a book, or listening to soothing music. Get the mind and body ready for sleep. This will make falling asleep easier. You will be able to transition into a deeper sleep. The routine should begin early enough that you are able to fall asleep at regular intervals. If you are unable to avoid stress, go back to those tips I just gave your earlier to deal with stress in your life.

- *Create a comfy sleep environment.* It should be dark, quiet, comfortable, and cool. Eye shades/masks and earplugs help block out distractions, such as a snoring partner. You could also go in a basement where it is quieter and cooler.

- *Take a supplement.* If you struggle with sleep following the other suggestions, you could also try two natural supplements called 5-HTP and Melatonin, popular sleep aids that help to boost serotonin levels, which improve mood and sleep.

- *Avoid caffeine in the evening.* Caffeine is a stimulant. Avoid having any within five hours of your bedtime. This may help improve sleep quality too!

The key is to experiment. What works for some might not work as well for others. It's important to find the sleep strategies that are right for you.

CHAPTER SIX

Remove 1 Common Food Allergen That Causes Bloating

One little-known food allergy that causes belly fat and bloating is still hot off the presses. Let me ask you a question. Are you allergic to gluten/wheat? If you are, a big belly is your first clue. There is a new condition called wheat allergy/gluten intolerance. There is more and more evidence that shows a large number of people are allergic to gluten (a protein found in wheat, barley, and rye), and its number one symptom is bloating and a distended belly. The condition is nicknamed "wheat belly" from the book *Wheat Belly* by William Davis, which is well worth reading.

A wheat allergy is not the same thing as gluten intolerance, though they are related. Wheat allergies can come early in life (as with a small child) and can be outgrown, or they can come late in life. The severity of the reaction to wheat varies according to a person's sensitivity. A wheat allergy often appears as intestinal distress (stomachaches, rashes/hives, vomiting, diarrhea, gas, constipation, and bloating). In contrast, gluten intolerance is a life-long autoimmune disease that involves the body attacking the lining of the small intestine, causing digestive distress, bloated belly, stomachache, and other serious symptoms.

While gluten intolerance and wheat allergy are different conditions, people who suffer from either of these conditions must avoid wheat, rye, and barley altogether; this includes spelt, bulgur, farina, and couscous—all forms of wheat. This is why gluten-free diets and cookbooks have become so popular! But here's what you need to know: Foods labeled as gluten-free are safe for both conditions! So if you have either of these conditions (wheat allergy or gluten intolerance), you're going to want to be shopping in the gluten-free aisles.

Understanding Gluten

Gluten is a special type of protein that is responsible for the elastic texture of dough. But not all foods from the grain family contain gluten. Examples of grains that do not have gluten include wild rice, corn, buckwheat, millet, quinoa, oats, and soybeans. These are great options if you have gluten intolerance. Gluten is not a naturally occurring protein in the human body. Studies have shown that it can cause general inflammation of the intestinal tract and can also damage the lining of the small intestine, making it difficult to absorb nutrients from foods.

Many people don't recognize gluten intolerance or food allergies in general because the symptoms are not the kinds of dramatic reactions that can land someone in the emergency room with hives or shortness of breath, like what happens to someone with a peanut allergy who has ingested peanuts. The reactions to gluten are much less dramatic but just as deadly. They play a huge role in chronic illness and weight issues.

Gluten reactions affect millions of people, but they are not easily diagnosed. The reaction is often delayed, causing symptoms anywhere from a few hours to several days after consumption. These delayed allergic reactions include weight gain, bloated belly, fluid retention, skin eruptions, fatigue, brain fog, irritable bowel syndrome, mood problems, headaches, sinus and nasal congestion, and muscle and joint pain or swelling. Some of the more common foods people are often allergic to are wheat, gluten, dairy, and peanuts. Eating foods you are allergic to causes inflammation, which ultimately leads to swelling and fluid retention. Getting rid of this fluid by reducing inflammation is a good thing and can really help you improve your health!

Eliminating food allergies is the foundation for feeling better and dealing with chronic symptoms. So how do you find out if you are allergic to wheat/gluten? To determine what foods you're allergic to, you can take a blood test for immunoglobulin G (IgG) antibodies to foods. This can be helpful but may not detect all food allergies.

I recommend my clients identify food allergies by the "process of elimination." I had one client totally clear up her acne and skin rashes this way. You get rid of all potential foods you think you may be allergic to (e.g., wheat and gluten) for three or four weeks. Then reintroduce them gradually, one at a time, to see how your system reacts to each one. Keep a food journal and take notes on how different foods affect how you feel or what symptoms they cause in your body. Write down what you eat, when you ate it, and how you felt for the next couple of days after you ate it.

For example, if you are trying to determine if you are allergic to wheat, you could eat a serving of Cream of Wheat at breakfast and maybe a sandwich with wheat bread for lunch. Then observe your body carefully for the next two to three days. Watch to see if the wheat triggers any symptoms such as fluid retention, bloated belly, constipation or diarrhea, headaches, runny nose, or joint pain. If you experience such reactions or symptoms after you reintroduce the food, do not continue to include that food in your diet. Instead, wait and retry again in another month or two. If you still react negatively, you should just remove them from your diet altogether or visit a dietitian or nutritionist specialized in managing food allergies.

Because the foods we're most allergic or sensitive to are the ones we eat daily and crave, avoiding these foods can initially be a challenge. You should expect withdrawal symptoms and cravings for those foods for three to four days. Additionally, any of the allergic reactions could worsen during that timeframe. However, after those few days, you will feel better and begin to experience a sense of wellbeing. Once you eliminate wheat/gluten, if that is what you are allergic to, your body can begin to heal and that bloated belly/fluid retention will go away.

⚜   ⚜   ⚜

Getting rid of belly fat requires a commitment to change: your thinking, your lifestyle, your mindset. It requires gaining new knowledge, and making some permanent changes in your life for the better!

Once again, congrats on making an investment in you. Belly fat is dangerously unhealthy, and you will be so much happier with slimmer, sexier abs. Measure your results and watch the inches melt away. I look forward to hearing from you!

Frequently Asked Questions (FAQs)

1. Can I use products/brands other than the ones you recommend?

Yes, that's totally up to you. I only recommend products that my peers, my clients, and I use that actually work. If you want to use something else, please do your research and due diligence because there are a lot of low-quality, ineffective products on the market.

2. Where is the best place to buy the products?

The majority of products are available online. You can view our website to order many of them at:

http://jjsmithonline.com/products/buy-products.html

Also, many of the products are sold at health-food stores or speciality stores, such as Vitamin Shoppe and Whole Foods.

3. Are agave syrup, honey, raw sugar, and brown sugar good alternatives to white sugar?

They are okay in moderation. They will still cause insulin spikes that result in fat storage in the body. Stevia is best if you're trying to lose belly fat—or body fat, for that matter. The way to judge sweeteners is to think about their glycemic index (GI), or how much they cause insulin spikes, because that determines how much they will also cause fat storage in the body. Stevia has a GI of 0, which is ideal; agave 20, honey about 30, brown sugar/raw sugar 65; and white refined sugar 80. That should give you some perspective on your best options for sweeteners that reduce body fat.

4. Is Truvia the same as stevia?

Truvia is made from the stevia plant, but some reports say it contains chemicals that can be damaging to the body. Also, due to the presence of the sugar alcohol erythritol in Truvia, you may experience digestive disruptions if you are sensitive to sugar alternatives. Your best bet is always an all-natural 100% Stevia extract. However, do your own research to determine if Truvia is acceptable to you. Many people have great success with Truvia.

5. I don't like the taste of stevia. Are there other options?

Every brand of stevia tastes different, so it's not the stevia but the brand. It's worth finding one you like if you seriously want to get rid of belly fat/body fat. I have four friends who use four different brands of stevia, and none of us likes the others' stevia because the tastes are that different. Try another brand.

6. I get a headache when I remove the seven foods. Is that normal?

You're experiencing detox symptoms. You should expect and welcome them because, although they can be unpleasant, they are signs of progress. Detox symptoms can include headaches, fatigue, intense cravings, gas, and irritability. These symptoms may last for a few days or a few weeks, depending upon how toxic or how dependent your body is on the seven foods. The process will seem difficult, but you will begin to feel better soon.

7. Are there any cereals that you recommend besides oatmeal?

Yes, the two best makers of cold and hot cereals are Bob's Red Mill and Ezekial 4:9. They both have numerous options and always use non-dairy milks, such as unsweetened almond milk, soymilk, etc.

8. What kind of salt or seasonings can I use?

Sea salt is slightly healthier, but you still need to use it in moderation. Try cayenne pepper, fresh peppers, onions, garlic, and natural herbs and seasonings. If you're used to using a lot of table salt, switch to sea salt and reduce your intake as a first step to reducing sodium.

9. I don't like plain water. Can I add Crystal Light to the water?

Very few people like plain water, but we understand it is necessary for a healthy, functioning body and critical for weight loss. Try adding some fresh lemon to your water.

Regarding Crystal Light, some of the flavors may use artificial sweeteners, which is one of the foods that we should be avoiding. Always check the label to see, as I've never used Crystal Light before. You have to make the call on which product brands are right for you.

10. Can I eat salted nuts and seeds as a snack? What are the best nuts to eat?

Raw and unsalted nuts and seeds are the healthiest. After that, roasted and unsalted are okay. But you rarely want to eat salted nuts and seeds. My favorite nuts and seeds are almonds, walnuts, pecans, pistachios, and sunflower seeds. However, there are many other healthy options.

11. I love pasta. Can I have whole-grain pasta, since I can't have white pasta?

Whole grain pasta is healthier than white pasta. You can eat it on occasion, but too much of it will slow your fat-burning. You're better off breaking your addiction to carbs, as that is a sugar addiction, before trying to reintroduce any type of pastas into your diet.

12. Can you take more than one supplement at a time?

You should take one supplement, or a maximum of two, to start or else you won't be able to determine which one is most effective for your body. Some supplements are more effective than others, so you don't want to begin them all at once. As a side note, if you do the green tea, you should try one of the quality green tea products that we mention in this book. Why take a green tea supplement/capsule, when you can drink and enjoy the health benefits of green tea!

13. Should I be concerned about the caffeine in green tea?

Two to three cups of tea per day is fine, but if you're sensitive to caffeine, then either avoid it altogether or don't drink it late in the afternoon or evening so it won't interrupt good-quality sleep. Green tea is better than black tea or coffee because its caffeine works in a different way. Green tea makes the body's own energy use more efficient, thereby improving vitality and stamina without your having to experience the up-and-down effect typically experienced with caffeine. This is due to the large amount of tannins in green tea that ensures that the caffeine is taken to the brain in only small amounts, which harmonizes the energies in the body.

14. What dosage should we use for the belly fat supplements?

Always follow the recommended dosage on the bottle or as recommended by your physician.

15. Can you do the liver cleansing and colon cleansing at the same time?

Yes, they work well together when done at the same time. As you work to cleanse the liver of toxins and impurities, the colon cleansing will ensure that the toxins are eliminated from the body as quickly as possible. This will help minimize detox symptoms, so you'll feel better sooner!

16. The Mag07 product (you recommended for colon cleansing) doesn't indicate how long to take it. What would you suggest?

For Mag07, if you've never done colon cleansing before, the first time should be an intensive cleansing dosage of three to five capsules at bedtime for seven to ten days. If your stool becomes too loose, it's not clinical diarrhea but rather the liquefying of toxins and waste in the digestive tract. However, if you don't like your stools so loose, you can reduce the dosage to two to four capsules per night. After the intensive cleansing, you can continue to use Mag07 at a maintenance dosage (once a week or once a month) to keep your digestive tract cleansed.

17. When I think of cleansing, I think of staying in the bathroom all day. Is this true? Should this be done on the weekend when I'm not at work?

No, the products I recommend have a mild cleansing effect. You will definitely move your bowels more often and more intensely, but you won't have to be glued to the bathroom!

APPENDIX B

Seven-Day Meal Plan

This seven-day meal plan will help get you started eating right to lose your belly fat. The recipes for these meals are included in Appendix C, which follows.

Day 1

Breakfast: Almond Butter Oatmeal

Lunch: Spinach Salad with Apples and Walnuts

Dinner: Almond-Crusted Baked Chicken and Candied Yams

Snacks: 1 red apple; lightly salted popcorn

Day 2

Breakfast: Cottage Cheese with Berries and Walnuts

Lunch: Navy Bean and Barley Soup with whole-grain crackers

Dinner: Veggie Burger, sautéed spinach in extra-virgin olive oil

Snacks: 1 cup of strawberries; unsweetened peanut butter with celery

Day 3

Breakfast: Granola Berry Parfait

Lunch: Tuna Salad with whole-grain crackers

Dinner: Black-Eyed Peas and Veggie-Stuffed Peppers

Snacks: 1 cup blueberries; 1 plain yogurt with berries

Day 4

Breakfast: Whole-Wheat Blueberry Pancakes

Lunch: Black Bean Quinoa Salad

Dinner: Baked Lemon Chicken, Garlic Mashed Turnips, Sautéed Tomatoes and Spinach

Snacks: 1 orange; 1 hard-boiled egg

Day 5

Breakfast: Basic Healthy Oatmeal with Toppings

Lunch: Caesar Salad with Chicken

Dinner: Marinated Veggie Stir-Fry with Brown Rice

Snacks: 1 green apple; lightly salted popcorn

Day 6

Breakfast: Cinnamon Granola

Lunch: Quinoa Veggie Salad

Dinner: Grilled Marinated Flank Steak with baked sweet potato and green salad

Snacks: 1 cup raspberries; 2 carrots

Day 7

Breakfast: Spinach and Tofu Scramble

Lunch: Old-Fashioned Chicken Noodle Soup with whole-wheat crackers

Dinner: Glazed Salmon and Collard Greens with Turkey Sausage

Snacks: 1 pear; unsweetened almond butter on celery

Appendix C

50 Lose-the-Belly-Fat Recipes

These recipes (on the following pages) are designed to help eliminate belly fat and bloating. Add as many of them as you can to your diet.

Cinnamon Granola

3 cups rolled oats

2 teaspoons cinnamon

¼ cup agave syrup

½ cup chopped walnuts

½ cup unsweetened applesauce

1. Preheat oven to 325°F.
2. Place oats, walnuts, and cinnamon in a bowl and mix.
3. Add applesauce and agave nectar and blend well.
4. Spread over parchment-lined baking sheet.
5. Bake for 45 to 60 minutes, stirring every 10 to 15 minutes so it doesn't burn.
6. Remove when it feels dry and has a golden-brown color.
7. Cool before serving.

Granola Berry Parfait

½ cup raspberries

½ cup blueberries

1 banana, sliced

1½ cups of granola

1 container of fat-free yogurt

Layer the banana, berries, yogurt, and granola in two tall glasses. Serve immediately.

Cottage Cheese with Berries and Walnuts

½ cup low-fat or nonfat cottage cheese

¼ cup fresh blueberries

¼ cup fresh strawberries, chopped

¼ cup walnuts

Place all ingredients into a bowl, mix, and serve.

Almond Butter Oatmeal

1 cup cooked rolled oats (cooked in unsweetened almond milk)

2 tablespoons almond butter

1 teaspoon cinnamon

1 tablespoon honey

> While the oats are still warm, combine all ingredients in a bowl and mix well until almond butter is blended.

Spinach Salad
with Apples and Walnuts

6 ounces of baby spinach, washed

½ cup walnuts

2 large green apples, cut into thin slices

2 tablespoons golden raisins

3 tablespoons red onion, chopped

2 tablespoons extra-virgin olive oil

2 tablespoon white-wine vinegar

1 tablespoon honey

½ teaspoon sea salt

½ teaspoon ground black pepper

3 ounces reduced-fat crumbled goat cheese

1. Toast the walnuts in a large nonstick skillet over medium heat, stirring every 3 to 4 minutes. Set aside on a plate to cool.

2. Whisk the oil, vinegar, honey, sea salt, and black pepper in salad bowl.

3. Stir in the onions, apples, and raisins; add spinach; toss to coat evenly.

4. Sprinkle on walnuts and goat cheese before serving.

Candied Yams

They taste just like Mama's candied yams but with healthier ingredients.

5 or 6 medium-sized yams

3 tablespoons stevia powder

1 tablespoon Earth Balance spread (non-dairy butter)

Lemon juice from half a lemon

1 tablespoon vanilla extract

Dash of cinnamon and nutmeg

1. Place yams, stevia, non-dairy butter, vanilla extract, and lemon juice in a skillet.
2. Slow-cook on low-medium heat
3. When yams are soft, remove mixture from heat, place in a bowl, and sprinkle with cinnamon and nutmeg.

Chicken and Brown Rice Soup

A healthier alternative to Chicken Noodle Soup

4 large chicken breasts

2 cups of cooked brown rice

3 teaspoons oregano

1 tablespoon extra-virgin olive oil

1 teaspoon garlic powder

1 large onion, chopped

2 large leeks, chopped

6 small carrots, peeled and sliced

2 parsnips, peeled and sliced

4 cups chicken broth

4 cups water

1. Sauté the onions, leeks, carrots, and parsnips for 6 to 7 minutes in the olive oil until the leeks and onions wilt.
2. Place vegetables in a large soup pot; add chicken broth, water, and herbs and simmer for 30 minutes.
3. Add chicken breast and simmer for an additional 30 minutes.

Navy Bean and Barley Soup

2 cans navy beans

3 large carrots

1 pound frozen peas

4 stalks celery

8 cups veggie stock

4 teaspoons fresh oregano

½ cup cooked barley

1. Place veggie stock, herbs, celery, carrots, and peas into the pot and bring to a boil.
2. Once the veggies are soft, add beans and cook long enough to warm them.
3. Put barley into a bowl and top with soup.
4. Add sea salt to taste.

Almond-Crusted Baked Chicken

3 medium chicken breasts

2 egg whites

1 cup of almonds

¼ cup parmesan cheese

1 teaspoon thyme

2 teaspoons oregano

1 teaspoon sea salt

1. Preheat oven to 350° F.
2. Place almonds, oregano, parmesan cheese, sea salt, and thyme into a food processor and process until well blended.
3. Place chicken on one plate, egg whites in a shallow bowl, and almond mixture on a second plate.
4. Gently roll each piece of chicken in egg whites, then in the almond mixture, and place on parchment-lined baking sheet.
5. Bake for about 30 minutes.

Veggie Burger

This is a great alternative to a beef burger, with delicious taste and flavor.

Burger Ingredients:

2 pounds cooked black beans (canned is fine)

1 cup whole-wheat flour

4 cups cooked brown rice

2 six-ounce packages of mushrooms

1 green pepper, diced

1 red pepper, diced

1 onion, diced

½ cup onion powder

½ cup garlic powder

1 cup nutritional yeast

¼ cup poultry seasoning

1 tablespoon sea salt

¼ cup basil leaves

1. In food processor, blend black beans and half of the mushrooms.
2. Place mixture into a bowl.

3. Chop the remaining mushrooms very finely and add to bowl.

4. Add remaining ingredients.

5. Form into a patty and cook over medium heat.

Tuna Salad

3 cans water-packed tuna

½ cup nonfat Greek yogurt

2 teaspoons lemon juice

1 carrot, grated

1 hard-boiled egg

1 small tomato

½ small white onion, minced

½ teaspoon dried dill

1 teaspoon dried parsley

¼ teaspoon Dijon mustard

½ teaspoon garlic powder

1 teaspoon agave

Dash of sea salt

Black pepper to taste

Mix all the ingredients together in one large bowl and serve.

Quinoa Pilaf

A healthy gluten-free meal that's very filling.

1 cup uncooked quinoa

1 cup uncooked red lentils

1 medium red bell pepper, chopped

¼ cup raisins

2 tablespoons extra-virgin olive oil

¼ cup orange juice (fresh squeezed is best)

¼ cup apple cider vinegar

2 cloves garlic, peeled and minced

2 tablespoons tamari soy sauce

1 teaspoon caraway seeds

½ teaspoon red pepper flakes

½ teaspoon sea salt to taste

½ cup roasted unsalted cashews, chopped

1. Rinse and cook quinoa in 2 quarts of water for 10 minutes.
2. Drain quinoa, place in a bowl, and let cool.
3. Add all other ingredients except cashews in a large bowl.
4. Add cashews when ready to eat.

Black-Eyed Peas and Veggie-Stuffed Peppers

A Creole-inspired meal that is mildly spicy with black-eyed peas, veggies, herbs, and spices.

4 large bell peppers, cut in half lengthwise

2 cans black-eyed peas, drained and rinsed

1 can diced tomatoes

1 cup diced carrots

2 jalapeños, sliced finely

1 medium yellow onion, finely chopped

2 tablespoons extra-virgin olive oil

4 garlic cloves, minced

2 dried bay leaves

1 teaspoon dried oregano

1 teaspoon dried basil

2 teaspoons paprika

3 sprigs of fresh thyme

1 teaspoon sea salt

¼ cup fresh parsley, chopped

1. Heat oven to 350°F and spray a 9x13 pan with olive oil.

2. Boil bell pepper halves in water for 5 minutes; drain and let cool.

3. Sauté onions, carrots, and jalapeño peppers over medium-high heat for 10 minutes. Add the garlic after about 5 minutes.

4. Add the other herbs, spices, and sea salt and sauté for another minute.

5. Add tomatoes and peas and stir; cover and simmer for 10 minutes; mix in parsley.

6. Remove bay leaves and thyme sprigs.

7. Place ½ cup of the veggie mixture into each pepper half.

8. Place the pepper halves into the 9x13 pan and bake for 25 minutes.

Black Bean Quinoa Salad

A great dish of beans, grains, and fruit that is healthy and flavorful.

1 can black beans

2 cups cooked quinoa

1 mango, peeled and diced

1 red bell pepper, diced

1 cup chopped green onions

1 cup chopped fresh parsley

2 tablespoons red wine vinegar

2 tablespoons grapeseed oil

¼ teaspoon sea salt

1. Combine the red pepper, green onions, mango, and parsley in a bowl.
2. Add the vinegar, grapeseed oil, and sea salt and stir.
3. Add the quinoa and stir.
4. Gently fold in the black beans.
5. Serve at room temperature or chilled.

Sautéed Tomatoes and Spinach

A healthy, tasty recipe of spinach and tomatoes sautéed to perfection.

2 plum tomatoes, seeded and diced

1 bunch of spinach (6 cups loosely packed)

2 tablespoons grapeseed oil

1 small onion, minced

3 garlic cloves, minced

2 teaspoons fresh ginger, sliced

½ teaspoon sea salt

Juice from ½ lemon

1. Heat a large skillet over medium-high heat and sauté the onions in the oil for 2 minutes.
2. Add ginger, garlic, and sea salt and sauté for 30 seconds.
3. Add tomatoes and sauté for about 2 minutes.
4. Add spinach and cook until wilted; add splashes of water so spinach doesn't burn.
5. Sprinkle in lemon juice and serve.

Green Leafy Stir-Fry

There's nothing healthier than green leafy veggies. And eating them will help you with weight loss, detoxification, and overall good health.

1 pound of dark leafy veggies (collards, kale, spinach, mustard greens, dandelion greens, etc.)

2 tablespoons peanut oil

3 cloves of garlic, minced

½ inch cube of ginger (grated)

1 tablespoon cooking sherry

2 teaspoons of soy sauce

1 teaspoon sesame oil

Pinch of raw sugar

1. Slice greens into 1-inch-wide sections; wash and dry.
2. Heat the peanut oil over medium-high heat in a nonstick skillet and add garlic and ginger.
3. Stir constantly for a few minutes or until stems begin to soften.

Braised Tofu

1 pound extra-firm tofu

¼ cup water

2 cloves garlic, minced

3 tablespoons fresh lemon juice

2 tablespoons soy sauce

Olive oil cooking spray

1. Preheat oven to 425°F or, if you have a separate broiler compartment, turn it on to preheat.
2. Press moisture out of tofu (you do not have to squeeze it, just press down on it).
3. Cut tofu into triangles (about 16).
4. Place all other ingredients in small bowl and mix.
5. Spray olive oil on an oven pan or baking sheet; dip each piece of tofu in the braising sauce and place on the pan/baking sheet.
6. Place pan or baking sheet in the oven or under broiler and bake or broil for 5 to 10 minutes until tofu is lightly browned.
7. Remove the pan and pour a few spoonfuls of braising sauce over the tofu; replace in oven for 3 more minutes.
8. Repeat one more time until tofu is golden brown.

Pea Soup

Fresh spring pea soup!

10 ounces of fresh or frozen peas

1 medium avocado, halved and pitted

1 cup water

1 cup unsweetened almond milk

2 tablespoons lime juice

½ teaspoon chili powder

Pinch of sea salt

Black pepper to taste

1. Blend all ingredients in a food processor until smooth
2. Heat and serve with black pepper.

Quinoa Veggie Salad

Quinoa is a healthy grain that tastes great with all kinds of veggies.

1 cup quinoa

2 cups water

2 small zucchinis, chopped

1 medium carrot, chopped

1 small red onion, chopped

2 tablespoons extra-virgin olive oil

2 small squash, chopped

Dash of salt (optional)

Juice from one lemon (optional)

1. Roast vegetables in oven at 300°F until tender.
2. Bring the quinoa and water to a boil in a medium pot, reduce heat, and simmer for 10 to 12 minutes until quinoa is fluffy.
3. Toss all ingredients together in a large bowl.
4. Serve warm or at room temperature with a dash of sea salt or fresh lemon juice to taste.

Baked Lemon Chicken

3 pounds of chicken breast

2 tablespoons extra-virgin olive oil

2 tablespoons chopped basil

¼ cup fresh lemon juice

1. Combine chicken, basil, lemon juice, and olive oil in a large bowl and toss together.
2. Refrigerate and let marinate for 2 hours.
3. Bake at 425°F for 50 to 60 minutes and serve.

Garlic Mashed Turnips

Mashed turnips make a great substitute for mashed potatoes. They are healthier and every bit as tasty.

3 cups turnips, diced

2 cloves garlic, chopped

Olive oil to taste

Sea salt to taste

1. Boil turnips and garlic for 15 minutes or until soft. Drain.
2. Mash turnips and garlic together in a bowl and add olive oil.
3. Add sea salt to taste.

Creamy Pea Soup

2 cups peas (fresh, canned, or frozen and thawed)

1 avocado

1½ cucumbers

2 tablespoons fresh lemon juice

2 garlic cloves

1 cup unsweetened almond milk

1. Place all ingredients in a food processor or blender and blend well.
2. Pour into a pan and heat.
3. Sprinkle with chopped parsley and serve.

Kale and Onion Soup

1 bunch kale, washed, stems removed, chopped

1 small onion, sliced

1 quart of vegetable broth

1. Place all ingredients into a soup pot and simmer for about 4 hours; let cool.
2. Separate solids from broth by using a strainer
3. Place onion and kale into a food processor and puree until creamy.
4. Recombine all ingredients and serve.

Basic Caesar Salad

1 head of romaine lettuce, torn into bite-size pieces

1 tablespoon fresh lemon juice

1 teaspoon apple cider vinegar

1 teaspoon dry mustard

1 teaspoon Worcestershire sauce

1 teaspoon anchovy paste

¼ cup extra-virgin olive oil

⅓ cup grated parmesan cheese

whole-wheat croutons (optional)

1. In a large salad bowl, whisk together the garlic, sea salt, oil, lemon juice, vinegar, mustard, Worcestershire sauce, and anchovy paste.

2. Add lettuce and toss to evenly coat.

3. Sprinkle with the parmesan cheese.

4. Add whole-wheat croutons (optional).

Marinated Veggie Stir Fry with Brown Rice

1 large onion, chopped

4 medium carrots, chopped

2 medium zucchinis, chopped

2 large red peppers, chopped

2 medium yellow squash, chopped

Marinade

3 tablespoons extra-virgin olive oil, divided

1/4 cup balsamic vinegar

1 teaspoon chopped oregano

1 garlic clove, minced

¼ teaspoon sea salt

½ teaspoon ground coriander

1/4 teaspoon ground cumin

½ teaspoon ground black pepper

1 teaspoon agave syrup

2 cups cooked brown rice

1. In a large bowl, combine 1 tablespoon oil, vinegar, oregano, garlic, coriander, cumin, sea salt, pepper, and agave syrup.

2. Add veggies, coat with marinade, and let stand for 30 minutes.

3. Drain the veggies and save the marinade.

4. Heat the remaining 2 tablespoons of oil in large skillet.

5. Cook the onion and carrots, stirring constantly for 5 to 7 minutes.

6. Add the zucchini and yellow squash, stirring constantly for another 2 to 3 minutes.

7. Add the bell peppers and cook for another minute, stirring constantly.

8. Add 2 to 3 tablespoons of remaining marinade to the veggies and stir constantly until veggies and marinade are hot, about 1 to 2 minutes more.

9. Serve over brown rice, if desired.

Grilled Marinated Flank Steak

1 pound flank steak

¼ cup red wine vinegar

¼ cup fresh lemon juice

2 tablespoons extra-virgin olive oil

2 tablespoons packed light brown sugar (or substitute a teaspoon of agave syrup)

2 tablespoons Dijon mustard

1 large garlic clove, minced

2 teaspoons fresh basil

1 teaspoon sea salt

Dash of fresh ground pepper

1. In a medium bowl, whisk together the vinegar, lemon juice, oil, sugar, mustard, garlic, sea salt, oregano, and hot pepper sauce until thoroughly combined.
2. Pour into a food storage bag, add the flank steak, and marinate overnight.
3. Grill the steaks on medium-high heat for 3 to 4 minutes on each side, depending on desired taste
4. Place the steaks on a plate, cover with aluminum foil, and let stand for 10 minutes.

Glazed Salmon

4 salmon fillets

¼ cup tamari soy sauce

2 tablespoons raw honey

1 tablespoon rice vinegar

1 tablespoon ground ginger

¼ teaspoon cayenne pepper

⅛ teaspoon ground pepper

1. In a large bowl, combine the soy sauce, honey, vinegar, ginger, cayenne, and black pepper.
2. Add the salmon and marinate in a food storage bag for 2 hours.
3. Preheat the broiler and place salmon on a broiler rack for 8 to 10 minutes, until flaky with a fork. Serve.

Pineapple Peppered Mahi-Mahi with Couscous

4 4-ounce boneless, skinless mahi-mahi fillets

1 cup whole-wheat couscous

2⅓ cups low-sodium chicken broth, divided

2 teaspoon extra-virgin olive oil

2 cups chopped fresh pineapple

1 red bell pepper, diced

2 tablespoon fresh chives, chopped

¼ teaspoon sea salt

fresh ground black pepper to taste

1. In a small saucepan, bring 1⅓ cups broth to a boil on high heat. Stir in couscous.
2. Remove from heat immediately, cover, and let sit for 5 minutes, until liquid is absorbed.
3. In a large skillet, heat olive oil on medium-high.
4. Season both sides of mahi-mahi with sea salt and black pepper. Add mahi-mahi to skillet and cook for 1 minute per side, until golden. Remove from pan and set aside.

5. Add pineapple and bell pepper to skillet and cook on medium-high for 2 minutes, until soft, stirring occasionally.

6. Stir in cooked couscous, remaining 1 cup broth, and chives; mix well.

7. Arrange mahi-mahi on top of couscous mixture, cover with foil and cook for 2 minutes, until mahi-mahi is tender and steaming under foil.

Mushroom Steak

4 5-ounce top loin steaks, all visible fat trimmed

1 pound of mushrooms cleaned, trimmed, and cut into ¼-inch slices

1 tablespoon olive oil

½ cup low-sodium beef broth

1 teaspoon low-sodium soy sauce

½ teaspoon sea salt

½ teaspoon black pepper

4 cloves garlic

1 tablespoon chopped fresh thyme

1. In a large nonstick skillet, heat oil on medium-high.
2. Season both sides of steaks with sea salt and pepper.
3. Add steaks to skillet and cook until done to taste (3 to 5 minutes per side). Let sit for 5 minutes.
4. Meanwhile, place same skillet on medium heat. Add garlic and cook, stirring, for 30 seconds.
5. Add mushrooms and thyme; cook, stirring occasionally, until mushrooms are tender, about 3 to 5 minutes.

6. Add broth and soy sauce, deglazing pan by scraping browned bits from bottom of skillet with a spoon or spatula.

7. Cook, stirring occasionally, until liquid is reduced to a thin layer, 1 to 2 minutes.

8. Serve steaks with mushroom mixture over top, dividing evenly

9. Garnish with additional thyme sprigs.

Seared Scallops with Vinaigrette Sauce

1 pound sea scallops

¾ cup soymilk

6 teaspoon olive oil, divided

2 cups fresh or frozen green peas

2 green onions, rinsed and thinly sliced

¼ teaspoon sea salt, divided in half

1 teaspoon fresh thyme leaves

1 teaspoon fresh lemon juice

2 teaspoons white wine vinegar

1 teaspoon minced fresh mint

½ teaspoon raw honey

1. Heat a skillet on medium-low and add 1 teaspoon oil and swirl to coat skillet.

2. Add green onions and 1/8 teaspoon salt and cook, stirring occasionally, until onions are softened and just starting to brown.

3. Add thyme, peas, and soymilk. Increase heat to medium and cook, stirring, until peas are heated through, about 5 minutes. Remove mixture from heat.

4. Scrape pea mixture into a blender and purée until smooth, adding a bit more milk to thin, if necessary.

5. Heat a large skillet on medium-high. Add 1 teaspoon oil and swirl to coat pan.

6. Add scallops, leaving a bit of space between each to prevent steaming. Sear scallops for about 3 minutes per side, until golden brown and barely firm to the touch. Place scallops on a plate.

7. In a small bowl, whisk together remaining 4 teaspoons of oil, lemon juice, vinegar, 1 teaspoon water, mint, honey, and remaining sea salt.

8. To serve, spoon ½ cup pea purée onto each of 4 plates and top with 4 scallops.

9. Spoon vinaigrette over top of scallops and serve.

Baked Halibut

2 5-ounce boneless, skin-on halibut fillets

1 teaspoon extra-virgin olive oil

1 large clove garlic, minced

2 teaspoons lemon zest

Juice from 1/2 lemon

1 tablespoon chopped parsley

Dash of sea salt

Dash of fresh ground black pepper

1. Preheat oven to 400°F.
2. In a large nonstick baking dish, add halibut, skin side down, and drizzle with oil.
3. Top with garlic, lemon zest, and 2 tablespoons of juice and parsley, dividing evenly; season with sea salt and pepper.
4. Bake for 12 to 15 minutes, until halibut flakes easily when tested with a fork.
5. Drizzle with remaining lemon juice and serve.

Collard Greens with Turkey Sausage

½ teaspoon chili powder

½ teaspoon paprika

¼ teaspoon sea salt

⅛ teaspoon of ground black pepper and cayenne pepper

3 medium shallots, thinly sliced

1 tablespoon extra-virgin olive oil, divided

2 lean fresh turkey sausages with casings removed

1 pound of collard greens, stems removed and leaves chopped

1. In a small bowl, mix together chili powder, paprika, salt, black pepper, and cayenne.
2. Heat 2 teaspoons oil in a large sauté pan on medium-high.
3. Add shallots and cook, stirring frequently, for 3 minutes, until softened.
4. Heat remaining olive oil in pan. Add sausage and cook, breaking up meat with a wooden spoon, for about 3 minutes, until browned.
5. Stir remaining spice mixture and collard greens into pan. Cover and cook for 2 minutes.
6. Remove lid, stir, and cook for 2 more minutes.
7. Add shallot mixture back to pan, stir, and cook for 1 more minute, until heated through.

Collard Green Stew with Black-Eyed Peas

8 cups collard greens, cleaned and chopped

1 can cooked black-eyed peas, rinsed and drained

1 can no-salt-added diced tomatoes

4 cups low-sodium vegetable broth

2 cups water

Black pepper, to taste

1. Bring broth and 2 cups water to a boil in a large saucepan on high heat.
2. Add collard greens, cover, and simmer for 15 minutes.
3. Add tomatoes and return to a simmer. Cover and cook until tomatoes are tender
4. Stir in black-eyed peas and simmer until heated through, about 2 minutes.
5. Season with pepper, to taste.

Baked Salmon in Spicy Lime-Cilantro Dressing

1 pound salmon fillet, skinned

1 chili pepper, seeded and cut into thin strips

⅓ cup fresh lime juice

2 green onions, sliced

1 cup packed fresh cilantro leaves, chopped

1 teaspoon canola oil

½ teaspoon sea salt

1. Preheat oven to 350°F.
2. Combine chili pepper, lime juice, onions, cilantro, oil, and salt in a food processor and purée.
3. Place salmon in a baking dish just large enough to fit fillet. Pour sauce from blender over salmon, turning fish to coat on both sides.
4. Bake, uncovered, until fish is cooked to your liking in center, 20 to 25 minutes depending on thickness of the fish.
5. To serve, slice fillet into pieces and spoon sauce over each portion.

Sweet Potato Fries

1 teaspoon fresh rosemary leaves, chopped

1 tablespoon extra-virgin olive oil

3 medium sweet potatoes, peeled

¼ teaspoon sea salt

1. Preheat oven to 425°F.
2. In a small bowl, combine rosemary and olive oil; set aside.
3. Scrub potatoes and cut each potato lengthwise into ½-inch slices; then, stacking 2 slices together, cut each into ½-inch strips.
4. In a large bowl, toss sweet potato strips with rosemary mixture until evenly coated.
5. Spread sweet potatoes on a large parchment-lined baking sheet in a single layer.
6. Bake for 30 to 35 minutes, flipping potatoes over halfway through baking time, until lightly browned.
7. Remove from oven, sprinkle with salt, and serve warm.

Spicy Orange Chicken with Brown Rice

4 boneless, skinless chicken breasts rinsed and patted dry

2 cups cooked brown rice

1 teaspoon chili powder

½ teaspoon ground cumin

1 teaspoon safflower oil

⅓ cup orange juice (no sugar added)

2 tablespoon pure maple syrup

1 tablespoon chopped chipotle chilies in adobo sauce

1 teaspoon orange zest

¼ packed cup chopped cilantro leaves

½ teaspoon sea salt

1. In a small bowl, combine chili powder, cumin, and ¼ teaspoon salt.
2. Heat oil in a large nonstick skillet to medium-high.
3. Season both sides of chicken with chili-cumin mixture and cook for 3 minutes per side or until no longer pink in center; remove from skillet and set aside.

4. Add orange juice and maple syrup to juice and bits left in skillet and cook for 1 minute to thicken slightly, stirring constantly.

5. Remove from heat, stir in chipotle chilies in adobo sauce and orange zest.

6. Return chicken to skillet and cook for 1 minute on medium-high, turning constantly.

7. In a medium bowl, combine brown rice, cilantro, and remaining sea salt.

8. Serve chicken over rice and spoon any excess glaze over top chicken pieces.

Salad with Lemon-Olive Oil Dressing

2 heads romaine lettuce or spinach leaves

2 cups mixed fresh herbs (such as cilantro, parsley, fennel, basil)

¼ cup chopped scallions

Dressing:

¼ cup extra-virgin olive oil

¼ cup lemon juice

⅛ teaspoon sea salt

Dash of ground black pepper

1. Tear lettuce into pieces and place in large salad bowl with fresh herbs and scallions.
2. In separate bowl, whisk together dressing ingredients.
3. Pour dressing over salad and toss to coat evenly.

Sautéed Yams

2 large yams, peeled and shredded

2 tablespoons extra-virgin olive oil

3 tablespoons lime juice

1 teaspoon ground nutmeg

2 tablespoon fresh ginger

1 red onion, minced

1. In large pan, sauté ginger and onion in olive oil over medium heat for 5 minutes.

2. Add shredded yams and lime juice and increase heat to medium-high. Stir continuously and sauté for 5 to 7 minutes until yams are soft.

3. Season with nutmeg and sea salt and pepper to taste.

4. Cook another 2 to 3 minutes.

Old-Fashioned Chicken Noodle Soup

1½ cup whole-wheat egg noodles

½ pound skinless chicken breast, cut into pieces

1 tablespoon Earth Balance buttery spread

¾ cup summer squash, chopped

¾ cup carrots, chopped

¼ cup celery, chopped

1 tablespoon cornstarch

½ cup water

2 cups low-sodium chicken broth

⅛ teaspoon stevia powder

1 teaspoon basil

1 tablespoon dry onion flakes

2 tablespoons chopped parsley

Sea salt and pepper to taste

1. Melt buttery spread in large pan over medium heat; add squash, carrots, and celery; sauté for 5 minutes

2. Combine cornstarch, water, stevia; add to vegetables and stir.

3. Add broth, basil, onion, sea salt, and pepper and bring to a boil.

4. Reduce heat to a simmer, cover, and cook 5 minutes.

5. Add noodles and chicken and bring to a boil.

6. Reduce heat, cover, and simmer 10 minutes.

7. Stir in parsley and serve.

Cabbage Seaweed Sauté

1 cup dried arame

4 cups water

½ cup small cabbage, thinly sliced

1 red onion, cut into wedges

3 medium carrots, cut into small pieces

2 tablespoons tamari soy sauce

1 teaspoon grapeseed oil

2 to 3 dashes plum vinegar

1 tablespoon toasted sesame oil

1. Soak arame in 4 cups of water for 15 minutes; drain and set aside.
2. In large skillet, sauté onion in grapeseed oil over medium heat for 3 minutes.
3. Add carrots and sauté another 2 to 3 minutes.
4. Add arame and heat through.
5. Remove from heat; add vinegar and sesame oil and serve warm.

Cucumber Tomato Salad

5 cups of heirloom tomatoes, chopped

2 small cucumbers, chopped

1 avocado, peeled, pitted, and chopped

¼ cup red onion finely chopped

¼ cup fresh basil, chopped

1 tablespoon red wine vinegar

2 tablespoons extra-virgin olive oil

1. Place tomatoes, cucumbers and avocado into a serving dish.
2. In a separate bowl, combine onion, basil, vinegar, oil, and salt and pepper to taste
3. Pour dressing over salad and serve.

Spinach Salad
with Vinaigrette Dressing

6 cups baby spinach, loosely packed

1 cup strawberries (stems removed)

¼ cup pumpkin seeds, toasted

Vinaigrette Dressing:

¼ cup extra-virgin olive oil

2 tablespoons red wine vinegar

1 teaspoon Dijon mustard

1 teaspoon agave syrup

Pinch of sea salt

1. Place spinach and ½ cup strawberries in a large bowl.
2. In a small bowl, whisk together dressing ingredients.
3. Pour vinaigrette over salad and toss to coat evenly.
4. Top with remaining seeds and strawberries.

Collards and Black-Eyed Peas

1 large bunch collard greens, chopped

1½ cups cooked black-eyed peas

2 garlic cloves, minced

2 tablespoons extra-virgin olive oil

½ onion, diced

Dash of apple cider vinegar

1. In large pot, sauté garlic and onion in olive oil over medium heat until soft.
2. Add collard greens and stir until wilted, adding extra water as needed to prevent from burning.
3. Add black-eyed peas and vinegar; continue cooking 3 to 4 minutes to heat through.
4. Season to taste with sea salt and pepper.

Whole-Grain Spaghetti with Crab Sauce

1 pound lump crabmeat

1 large tomato, chopped

4 ounces whole-grain spaghetti

1 bell pepper, cut into thin strips

1 red onion, cut into wedges

1 zucchini, sliced

2 garlic cloves

¼ cup extra virgin olive oil

¼ cup fresh basil

¼ cup grated parmesan cheese

1. Pre-heat oven to 425°F..
2. Combine the peppers, onion, garlic, and zucchini in a 9x9- inch pan.
3. Sprinkle 2 tablespoons of olive oil and toss to evenly coat.
4. Roast for 15 minutes until veggies are browned.
5. Prepare the pasta per the package instructions; set aside half a cup of the cooking liquid before draining.

6. Combine the roasted vegetables, pasta, tomato, basil, and crab in a large bowl and toss to coat evenly.

7. Slowly add the pasta cooking liquid to moisten, as needed.

8. Sprinkle with parmesan cheese.

Scallops with Lemon Sauce

1½ pounds of sea scallops, washed and dried

¼ cup fresh parsley leaves

2 tablespoons fresh lemon juice

¼ cup extra-virgin olive oil

1 garlic clove, minced

½ teaspoon sea salt

¼ teaspoon ground pepper

1. Combine the lemon juice, parsley, garlic, sea salt, and pepper in a small bowl.
2. Whisk the olive oil into combined ingredients and set it aside.
3. Coat a pan with cooking spray over medium-heat.
4. Sprinkle sea salt and pepper on scallops, add to pan, and sauté for 2 to 3 minutes on each side.
5. Spoon the sauce over scallops and serve.

Pork Tenderloin with Herbs and Capers

1 pound pork tenderloin, trimmed of fat

1 medium red onion, sliced

1 tablespoon fresh rosemary, minced

2 teaspoons extra virgin olive oil

¼ teaspoon sea salt

¼ teaspoon ground pepper

1 cup of capers

1. Pre-heat oven to 375°F.
2. Place the pork, red onion, and rosemary on a baking sheet covered with aluminum foil; add oil, pepper, and sea salt and rub onto pork to coat.
3. Roast for 20 minutes.
4. Scatter the capers over the onions and pork and toss to combine; return to oven and roast for another 15 minutes.
5. Let stand for 10 to 15 minutes before slicing.

Olive Oil and Lemon Dressing

A healthy homemade salad dressing.

⅓ cup extra-virgin olive oil

¼ cup lemon juice

3 cloves of garlic chopped finely

1 teaspoon dried oregano

1 teaspoon dried marjoram

1 teaspoon dried basil

½ teaspoon sea salt

dash of pepper

1. Whisk all ingredients together.
2. Close tightly in a container and refrigerate for 2 hours before serving.

Apple Cider Vinaigrette Dressing

3 tablespoons apple cider vinegar

6 tablespoons extra-virgin olive oil

1 tablespoon honey

Pinch of sea salt

1. Whisk all ingredients together
2. Close tightly in a container and refrigerate for 2 hours until serving.

Old-Fashioned Carrot Cake

3 cups almond flour

1 cup chopped walnuts

1 cup raisins

3 cups grated carrots

5 large eggs

½ cup agave syrup

2 teaspoons sea salt

1 teaspoon baking soda

1 tablespoon ground cinnamon

1 teaspoon ground nutmeg

¼ cup grapeseed oil

1. Preheat oven to 325°F.
2. Grease two 9-inch cake pans with grapeseed oil and dust with almond flour.
3. Combine almond flour, sea salt, cinnamon, nutmeg, and baking soda in a large bowl.
4. In medium bowl, whisk together the grapeseed oil, agave syrup, and eggs.
5. Mix both the dry and wet ingredients together and then fold in carrots, walnuts and raisins.

6. Pour the batter into the two pans and bake for 30 to 35 minutes until inserting a toothpick in the center of cake comes out clean.

7. Let bread cool for about 1 hour and then it is ready to serve.

Banana Cake

1 cup mashed bananas (about 2 medium bananas)

½ cup chopped walnuts

3 cups whole-wheat pastry flour

1½ teaspoons stevia powder

4¼ teaspoons baking powder

¼ teaspoon sea salt

3 eggs, separated

1 cup soymilk

6 tablespoons canola oil

2½ teaspoons vanilla extract

1. Preheat oven to 350°F.
2. Place dry ingredients into a bowl and mix.
3. Beat egg whites in a separate bowl until stiff and set aside.
4. Stir together egg yolks, soymilk, canola oil, vanilla extract, and banana.
5. Add the dry ingredients and beat to combine.
6. Fold in beaten egg whites.
7. Pour mixture into an oiled cake pan dusted with flour and bake for 25 to 30 minutes.
8. Let cool for 10 minutes, and sprinkle nuts on top.

Homemade Butter Pecan Ice Cream

This recipe requires the use of an ice cream maker.

1½ cups of pecan pieces

2 cups coconut milk

1¼ cups cashew milk

½ cup agave syrup

7 tablespoons Earth Balance buttery spread, divided

2 teaspoon vanilla extract

½ teaspoon guar gum

¼ teaspoon sea salt

1. Spread pecans on a baking sheet and toast in oven at 350°F.
2. Place 2 tablespoons of buttery spread with ¼ teaspoon of sea salt into a bowl and set aside.
3. Blend coconut milk, cashew milk, agave syrup, remaining buttery spread, vanilla extract, and guar gum in a food processer until creamy and smooth.
4. Place in freezer for 1 hour.
5. Pour into ice cream machine and churn until soft.
6. Mix in pecans and serve.

Homemade Strawberry Ice Cream

This recipe requires the use of an ice cream maker.

2 cups strawberries

1½ cups coconut milk

1 cup cashew milk

½ cup agave syrup

2 teaspoons vanilla extract

1 teaspoon lemon juice

½ teaspoon guar gum

1. Place all ingredients into a blender and blend until creamy and smooth.
2. Place in freezer for 1 hour.
3. Pour into ice cream machine and churn until soft.
4. Top with fresh strawberries and serve.

About the Author

Bestselling author JJ Smith is a certified nutritionist and weight-loss expert, passionate relationship/life coach, and inspirational speaker. She has been featured on *The Steve Harvey Show*, *The Montel Williams Show*, *The Jamie Foxx Show*, and *The Michael Baisden Show*. JJ has appeared on the NBC, FOX, CBS, and CW Network television stations, as well as in the pages of *Glamour*, *Essence*, *Heart and Soul*, and *Ladies Home Journal*. Since reclaiming her health, losing weight, and discovering a "second youth" in her forties, JJ Smith has become the voice of inspiration to those who want to lose weight, be healthy, and get their sexy back! JJ Smith provides lifestyle solutions for losing weight, getting healthy, looking younger, and improving your love life! To learn more, check out www.JJSmithOnline.com.

JJ has dedicated her life to the field of healthy eating and living. Her passion is to educate others and share with them the natural remedies to stay slim, restore health, and look and feel younger. She has studied many philosophies of natural healing and learned from some of the great teachers of our time. After studying and applying knowledge about how to heal the body and lose weight, JJ went on to receive several certifications—one as a certified nutritionist and another as a certified weight-management expert. JJ received her certification as a nutritionist from the Institute of Holistic Healing. She received her certification as a weight-management specialist from the National Exercise and Sports Trainers Association

(NESTA). She is also a member of the American Nutrition Association (ANA).

JJ holds a B.A. in mathematics from Hampton University in Virginia. She continued her education by completing The Wharton Business School Executive Management Certificate program. She currently serves as vice president and partner at Intact Technology, an IT consulting firm in Greenbelt, Maryland. JJ was the youngest African American to become a vice president at a Fortune 500 company. Her hobbies include reading, writing, and deejaying.

To learn more, check out www.JJSmithOnline.com.

Lose Weight Without Dieting or Working Out!

www.JJSmithOnline.com

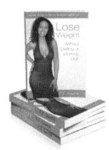 Want to lose weight without counting calories, starving yourself, giving up your favorite foods, or eating bland packaged foods? Would you like to look and feel younger and healthier than you have in years without diets and exercise? If you've answered yes to these questions, this book is for you! JJ Smith's revolutionary system teaches proven methods for permanent weight loss that anyone can follow, no matter their size, income level, or educational level. And the end result is a healthy, sexy, slim body.

You will learn how to....

✓ **Detoxify the body for fast weight loss**

✓ **Drop pounds and inches fast, without grueling workouts or starvation**

✓ **Lose up to 15 pounds in the first three weeks**

✓ **Shed unwanted fat by eating foods you love, including carbs**

✓ **Get rid of stubborn belly fat**

✓ **Trigger your 6 fat-burning hormones to lose weight effortlessly**

✓ **Eat foods that give you glowing, radiant skin**

✓ **Eat so you feel energetic and alive every day**

✓ **Get physically active without exercising**

This is your last stop on the way to a new fit and healthy you! Look and feel younger than you have in years.
Create your best body—NOW